James H. Elzerman
703 First Ave.
Morris, Illinois 60450
815-942-2104

TREATMENTS FOR THE ALZHEIMER PATIENT: THE LONG HAUL

Lissy F. Jarvik, M.D., Ph.D., is Professor, Department of Psychiatry and Biobehavioral Sciences, University of California, Los Angeles; Chief, Section on Neuropsychogeriatrics, UCLA Neuropsychiatric Institute and Hospital; and Chief, Psychogeriatric Unit, West Los Angeles Veterans Administration Medical Center, Brentwood Division. Her Ph.D. is in psychology from Columbia University, and her M.D. degree from Case Western Reserve University. Dr. Jarvik's major research interest has been the psychobiology of aging, particularly human genetics (including twin and family studies as well as studies of chromosomes and cell motility), mental functioning, depression and dementia (especially of the Alzheimer type), and geriatric psychopharmacology. She is author of over 200 articles on these subjects and has edited close to a dozen books. She serves on numerous editorial boards and is founding coeditor of the new publication *Alzheimer Disease and Associated Disorders—An International Journal*. As an expert in her field, Dr. Jarvik was invited in 1983 to testify at the first Congressional Hearing devoted exclusively to Alzheimer's disease. She is currently a member of the Board of Directors and the Medical and Scientific Advisory Board of the Alzheimer's Disease and Related Disorders Association (ADRDA) and, in recent years, has served on the NIMH National Advisory Health Council and the Alzheimer's Disease Task Force for the State of California.

In 1986 Dr. Jarvik received three major awards: the Jack Weinberg Memorial Award for Geriatric Psychiatry from the American Psychiatric Association; the Robert W. Kleemeier Award for Outstanding Research in the Field of Aging from the Gerontological Society of America; and the Edward B. Allen Award to a Scientist for Special Contribution to the Field of Geriatric Psychiatry from the American Geriatrics Society.

Carol Hutner Winograd, M.D. (Boston University), is Assistant Professor of Medicine (Gerontology), Stanford University School of Medicine; Director, Clinical Activities, Geriatric Research, Education and Clinical Center, Palo Alto Veterans Administration Medical Center; and Director of the Geriatric Clinic and the Inpatient Geriatric Consultation Service. Dr. Winograd's major scholarly interests are in Alzheimer's disease and geriatric health care delivery. She was a consultant to the Alzheimer's Disease Task Force for the state of California and is studying aspects of medical correlates of Alzheimer's disease. The recipient of a "Geriatric Medicine Academic Award" from the National Institute on Aging, she is the author of numerous articles and book chapters on geriatric health care delivery, Alzheimer's disease, and clinical geriatrics, has served on peer review panels, and is a reviewer for several journals in geriatric medicine. Dr. Winograd is a member of the editorial board of *Alzheimer Disease and Associated Disorders—An International Journal* and is Chairperson of the Public Policy Committee of the American Geriatrics Society.

Treatments for the Alzheimer Patient: The Long Haul

Lissy F. Jarvik, M.D., Ph.D
Carol Hutner Winograd, M.D.
Editors

SPRINGER PUBLISHING COMPANY
New York

*To all those Alzheimer patients
who have taught us what we know
about this devastating disease.*

Springer Publishing Company, Inc.
536 Broadway
New York, NY 10012

88 89 90 91 92 / 5 4 3 2 1

Library of Congress Cataloging-in-Publication Data

Treatments for the Alzheimer patient.

  Bibliography: p.
  Includes index.
  1. Alzheimer's disease—Treatment. I. Jarvik,
Lissy F. II. Winograd, Carol Hutner. [DNLM:
1. Alzheimer's Disease—therapy. WM 220 T7847]
RC523.T74   1988   616.8'3   87-37651
ISBN 0-8261-6000-X

Printed in the United States of America

Contents

Foreword

An entire lifetime has passed since Dr. Alois Alzheimer (1907) described the occurrence of senile plaques and neurofibrillary tangles in the brain of a woman who had originally presented with symptoms of paranoid delusions and erratic behavior. Individuals not yet born at that time are now the victims of the mind-crippling affliction that bears his name.

It has only been in the last decade, with the increasingly rapid growth of the older population and a corresponding increase in gerontologic studies, that serious steps have been taken toward understanding this condition. Until recently, senility of this type was felt to be an inevitable, untreatable deterioration related to aging. With raised consciousness, we now have a very different approach to the problem of an individual with impaired memory, altered intellectual abilities, and/or behavioral or emotional dysfunction.

In a comprehensive fashion, encompassing diagnosis, treatment and behavioral management, family assessment and support, and community involvement, we focus on Alzheimer's and related disorders as diseases that can be helped, rather than as hopeless conditions. We enlist public and political assistance and encourage research and training. This volume brings together an exceedingly knowledgeable group of people who are teachers and leaders in these efforts. Their varied points of view and experience make this collection especially valuable.

The campaign against Alzheimer's disease is ongoing. Although the cause and cure for this devastating illness remain mysteries, we are developing a growing understanding of its manifestations and an armamentarium of treatment and coping strategies. The struggle is an arduous one, a long haul, but we continue with the hope that a future will come when Alzeheimer's disease will no longer rob people of their lives and dreams.

ELLIOT STEIN, M.D.
President
American Association for
Geriatric Psychiatry

Prologue: The Present— Some Concerns

Alzheimer's disease is one of the critical diseases of the twentieth century. Often cited as the fourth most common cause of death in the United States today, Alzheimer's disease is a relative newcomer to the health care scene. It emerged from obscurity nearly seven decades after the first case report was published (Alzheimer, 1907) to become a household word in the Western world. Ironically, it is the triumphs of modern medicine that have brought this disease to such prominence. As advances in medicine have enabled vast numbers of people to survive to the biblical threescore years and ten, the prevalence of this degenerative disease afflicting primarily the elderly has soared. In coming decades, the ever-increasing number of those who will succumb may produce overwhelming health care, social, psychological, and economic consequences. Finding means of prevention and/or cure offers our only hope.

In recent years, research into possible etiologies of Alzheimer's disease has shown promise, yet funding for both research and treatment has been—and remains—grossly inadequate. In an era of shrinking national resources, policy makers are reluctant to devote large sums of money to the old. While underfunding is common in health and human service areas, special issues may intensify the problems of funding research in Alzheimer's disease. For example, until recently, the number of persons afflicted appeared to be relatively small, and the public was uninformed. Further, elderly people in our society are often devalued and avoided, possibly because their predicaments arouse feelings of guilt and anxiety in the rest of us.

The treatment of Alzheimer's disease is also impeded by a sense of "therapeutic nihilism," engendered by the fact that there is currently no cure for this catastrophic illness. Families of Alzheimer patients are

ix

frequently told, "Your wife (husband, brother, sister, mother, father) has Alzheimer's disease; there is nothing we can do."

The intention of this book is to challenge such therapeutic nihilism, to distinguish treatment from cure, and to encourage treatment of Alzheimer patients and their caregivers. In doing so, we follow medical tradition: physicians routinely treat patients with diseases for which there are no cures. Patients with cancer, multiple sclerosis, or Lou Gehrig's disease receive treatment and medical attention even though there is no cure for their maladies. Alzheimer patients deserve no less. Although, to date, drug therapies aimed at reversing the cognitive decline have proven largely ineffective, there are effective treatments for many of the symptoms of Alzheimer's disease. The purpose of this book is to provide a compendium of clinical wisdom regarding such treatments.

This volume grew out of a two-part symposium presented at the annual meeting of the Gerontological Society of America in November 1985. The contributors were kind enough to transform their spoken remarks into written form and update them for purposes of publication. The book is geared to health professionals in a variety of disciplines, but we have also attempted to make it accessible to lay persons working with, caring for, or interested in Alzheimer patients.

We have tried to cover the major areas impinging on treatment issues, but as with any book, space constraints necessitate limitations. Specifically, we omitted legal aspects germane to the Alzheimer patient (such as guardianship, conservatorship, and estate planning). Laws vary from state to state; thus, we recommend that professionals and caregivers desiring legal information contact local or state resources, such as chapters of the Alzheimer's Disease and Related Disorders Association (ADRDA), for advice and referral to attorneys specializing in dementing disorders.

Another area warranting more attention than we have been able to give is the subjective experience of caregivers. We recognize the need for the voices of caregivers to be heard by policy makers as well as health and social service professionals. In the one chapter written by a caregiver, James Reveley eloquently describes his experience as the husband of an Alzheimer patient. Mr. Reveley's burden is lightened somewhat by the economic resources available to him and by the skills and contacts he gained as a business executive. What is missing in this volume are the voices of the thousands of caregivers whose life position and economic status permit them neither sufficient support (emotional or economic) nor adequate respite to help them cope with this crippling disease. But various chapters in this book, though written by professionals, do consider some of the enormous problems faced by caregivers of Alzheimer patients.

As we reach the end of the twentieth century, the impact of Alzheimer's disease will necessitate allocation of substantial resources. Funding is needed, not only for basic research to determine its causes and explore means of prevention and cure, but also for applied research to enable us to deliver available treatments more efficiently and humanely than is the current norm. We need increased understanding of the potential usefulness of each element in the health care delivery system: home care as well as outpatient, hospital, respite, and long-term institutional care. What innovations in use of treatment settings, medical interventions, and behavior-management techniques can lessen the manifestations of Alzheimer's disease? What training, team work, and interdisciplinary approaches can enhance health care delivery to Alzheimer patients and their caregivers? What public policies are needed to preserve the physical, emotional, and economic well-being of caregivers? As life-preserving technology advances, so, too, does the need to address ethical questions, such as how long, under what conditions, and by whose choice life should be sustained.

Changes in family lifestyle—such as the rising divorce rate, declining fertility in some ethnic and socioeconomic groups, increasing number of women in the workforce, accelerating geographic mobility, decreasing neighborhood stability, and reduced family proximity—are bound to have profound consequences for Alzheimer patients. These changes create additional dilemmas requiring research and shifts in public policy. Thus, we must prepare now to care for the number of Alzheimer victims, especially women, who will not have family caregivers.

In the current political climate, major policy changes are unlikely, yet major policy changes are essential if we are to provide needed services to Alzheimer patients and their families. The reimbursement policy is one area that requires change. At present, services provided by team members who are not physicians are often not covered by Medicare. But only through use of multidisciplinary (and multiskill-level) teams can optimal treatment be rendered to Alzheimer patients and their caregivers. And, eventually, such treatment will also prove most cost-effective. At present, reimbursement for physician services rewards high-tech procedures rather than cognitive skills (e.g., clinical assessment and ongoing primary care), while the long-term care needed by so many Alzheimer (and other elderly) patients remains generally nonreimbursable by either government or private insurance. Even those few families wealthy enough and knowledgeable enough to manipulate bureaucratic systems must expend great effort to provide appropriate care for their afflicted loved ones. Moreover, most families with an Alzheimer patient are not wealthy or sophisticated in the workings of bureaucracies. Afflicted families are likely to be middle-income or poorer; the patient may live alone and lack supportive family members. Although the very poor may have access to federal and state assistance programs, inadequate as they are, the large majority of patients and families fall between the cracks. They have enough money to be ineligible for subsidies, but not enough money, resources, or knowledge of the assistance systems to provide adequate care.

Alzheimer's disease is devastating, but with improvements in public policy and research funding, the future holds potential for significant breakthroughs in understanding, treatment, and prevention of this twentieth-century scourge. It is our hope that this book will not only provide encouragement to practitioners to treat, but also that it will stimulate research aimed both at improving treatment modalities and at uncovering the secrets of Alzheimer's disease. Perhaps by the twenty-first century, Alzheimer's disease will join the ranks of truly curable conditions.

In the meantime, our goal for this book is to make available to health professionals, families, and other caregivers up-to-date information about treatment options. In this way, perhaps we can narrow the gap between the knowledge base of leaders in the field and that of the public at large. We hope that in some small way this book will help ease the burden of Alzheimer's disease borne by the victims, their loved ones, and their caregivers.

Carol Hutner Winograd, M.D.
Lissy F. Jarvik, M.D., Ph.D.

Acknowledgments

The editors wish to thank Hoechst-Roussell Pharmaceuticals Inc., Somerville, NJ; The Sandoz Corporation, East Hanover, NJ; Smith Kline and French Laboratories, Philadelphia, PA; and Warner-Lambert Company, Ann Arbor, MI for their support. We also wish to thank Susan Baram, Nancy Lei, and Pat Murdo for their editorial assistance and patience. Their carefulness and critical thinking were vital in completing this book. Thanks also to Peggy Hefter, Elizabeth Moore, Martha Morrell, and Bonny Obrig for their assistance in preparing the manuscripts. To our scientific reviewers—Joseph Barbaccia, M.D., James E. Birren, M.D., Leon J. Epstein, M.D., Ph.D., Paul Haber, M.D., Dolores Gallagher, Ph.D., Vita Kolodny, R.N., Eric Larson, M.D., Steven S. Matsuyama, Ph.D., Carl Salzman, M.D., Gary W. Small, M.D., Joanne Steuer, Ph.D., Larry W. Thompson, Ph.D., and T. Franklin Williams, M.D.—we are grateful for their scholarly critiques and comments. And most of all we wish to express our gratitude to Barbara Haber, the editors' editor, whose intelligence, perceptive comments, and writing skills enormously enhanced the quality of this book. Her standards of excellence were invaluable in enabling this book to come to fruition. We cannot thank her enough.

The editors wish to acknowledge the following grant support: NIMH Research Grant MH-40041, Subproject #4, NIH-NIA Research Grant 5K08 AG00246, and the Veterans Administration for Dr. Winograd; NIMH Research Grant MH 36205 and the Veterans Administration for Dr. Jarvik.

The opinions expressed herein are those of the authors and not necessarily those of the Veterans Administration.

Contributors

Elaine M. Brody, M.S.W. Adjunct Associate Professor of Social Work in Psychiatry, University of Pennsylvania; Associate Director of Research, Philadelphia Geriatric Center, Philadelphia, PA.

Irene Burnside, R.N., M.S. Associate Professor, San Jose State University, San Jose, CA.

Robert N. Butler, M.D. Brookdale Professor and Chairman, Gerald and May Ellen Ritter Department of Geriatrics and Adult Development, Mount Sinai Medical Center, New York, NY; Co-director, Alzheimer's Disease Research Center, National Institute on Aging.

Christine K. Cassel, M.D. Chief, Section of General Internal Medicine, Division of the Biological Sciences, Department of Medicine, The Pritzker School of Medicine; Director, Center on Aging, Health and Society, The University of Chicago, Chicago, IL.

Gene D. Cohen, M.D., Ph.D. Clinical Professor of Psychiatry, Georgetown University; Director, Program on Aging, National Institute of Mental Health, Rockville, MD.

Jonathan O. Cole, M.D. Lecturer in Psychiatry, Harvard Medical School; Chief, Psychopharmacology Program, McLean Hospital, Belmont, MA.

James L. Fozard, Ph.D. Associate Scientific Director for the Baltimore Longitudinal Study of Aging, National Institute on Aging, Gerontology Research Center, Baltimore, MD.

Mary Kane Goldstein, M.D. Assistant Clinical Professor of Medicine (Family Medicine), Stanford University School of Medicine; Staff Physician, Geriatric Research, Education and Clinical Center, Veterans Administration Medical Center, Palo Alto, CA.

Lissy F. Jarvik, M.D., Ph.D. Professor, Department of Psychiatry and Biobehavioral Sciences, University of California at Los Angeles; Chief, Psychogeriatric Unit, West Los Angeles Veterans Administration Medical Center, Brentwood Division, Los Angeles, CA.

Barbara Katzman, B.A. Public Affairs Specialist, National Institute on Aging, National Institutes of Health, Bethesda, MD.

Alan M. Kennedy, B.S. Program Analyst, Patient Treatment Service, Veterans Administration Central Office, Washington, DC.

Asenath LaRue, Ph.D. Associate Professor, Department of Psychiatry and Biobehavioral Sciences, Neuropsychiatric Institute and Hospital, Center for the Health Sciences, University of California, Los Angeles.

Mary Jane Lucas-Blaustein, R.N.,C. Assistant Professor, Psychiatry and Behavioral Sciences, The Johns Hopkins University School of Medicine, Baltimore, MD.

John H. Mather, M.D. Associate Executive Director for Medical and Research Affairs, Paralyzed Veterans of America, Washington, DC.

Edwin J. Olsen, M.D. Associate Professor of Clinical Psychiatry/Vice Chairman, Department of Psychiatry, Chief of Division of Geriatric Psychiatry, University of Miami, School of Medicine; Assistant Chief and Medical Director for Geriatrics and Extended Care, Director, Development and Management Service, Veterans Administration Central Office, Washington, DC.

James B. Reveley, B.A. Cofounder and former Vice President and Treasurer, Alzheimer's Disease and Related Disorders Association–Rochester Chapter, Rochester, NY.

Barry W. Rovner, M.D. Assistant Professor, Psychiatry and Behavioral Sciences, The Johns Hopkins University School of Medicine, Baltimore, MD.

Janet S. Sainer, M.S.W. Commissioner, New York City Department for the Aging, New York, NY.

Andrew Satlin, M.D. Instructor in Psychiatry, Harvard Medical School, Assistant Director of Geriatric Psychiatry, McLean Hospital, Belmont, MA.

Elliott Stein, M.D. President, American Association for Geriatric Psychiatry, Miami, FL.

Larry E. Tune, M.D. Professor, Psychiatry and Behavioral Sciences, The Johns Hopkins University School of Medicine, Baltimore, MD.

T. Franklin Williams, M.D. Director, National Institute on Aging, National Institutes of Health, Bethesda, MD.

Carol Hutner Winograd, M.D. Assistant Professor of Medicine (Gerontology), Stanford University School of Medicine; Director of Clinical Activities, Geriatric Research, Education and Clinical Center, Palo Alto Veterans Administration Medical Center, Palo Alto, CA.

PART I
Clinical Care

1

The Physician and the Alzheimer Patient

Carol Hutner Winograd

DEFINITION AND DIAGNOSIS OF ALZHEIMER'S DISEASE

Alzheimer's disease is a disorder with protean manifestations. No single sign or symptom is diagnostic of the disease. Alzheimer's disease is one of several dementias defined by the American Psychiatric Association (1987). (See Table 1.1.) The diagnosis of Alzheimer's disease is essentially a clinical process, including a complete history, physical examination, formal neurologic examination, and mental-status testing. Because symptoms mimicking dementia frequently result from medication side effects, a full drug history, including both prescription and nonprescription drugs, is an essential part of the initial evaluation. Clinical information given by the patient must be corroborated by family and others who know the patient well. For the purposes of discussion in this book, patients who have a clinical syndrome consistent with the *DSM-III-R* criteria (Table 1.1) and whose history, physical findings, and laboratory evaluation are consistent with Alzheimer's disease are said to have this disorder.

The typical history reveals a gradual onset of global cognitive decline, usually measured in months to years. Age at onset ranges from the fifth to the eighth or ninth decades. Patients whose symptoms begin before age 65 are said to have presenile dementia, whereas those over 65 are said to have senile dementia. Because the symptoms and pathology

Drugs are listed by both brand name and generic name in the Drug Index.

TABLE 1.1 DSM-III-R Diagnostic Criteria for
Primary Degenerative Dementia of the Alzheimer Type

 I. Demonstrable evidence of impairment in short- and long-term memory. Impairment in short-term memory (inability to learn new information) may be indicated by inability to remember three objects after five minutes. Long-term memory impairment (inability to remember information that was known in the past) may be indicated by inability to remember past personal information (e.g., what happened yesterday, birthplace, occupation) or facts of common knowledge (e.g., past Presidents, well-known dates).

 II. At least one of the following:
   A. impairment in abstract thinking, as indicated by inability to find similarities and differences between related words, difficulty in defining words and concepts, and other similar tasks
   B. impaired judgment, as indicated by inability to make reasonable plans to deal with interpersonal, family, and job-related problems and issues
   C. other disturbances of higher cortical function, such as aphasia (disorder of language), apraxia (inability to carry out motor activities despite intact comprehension and motor function), agnosia (failure to recognize or identify objects despite intact sensory function), and "constructional difficulty" (e.g., inability to copy three-dimensional figures, assemble blocks, or arrange sticks in specific designs)
   D. personality change, i.e., alteration or accentuation of premorbid traits

III. The disturbance in I and II significantly interferes with work or usual social activities or relationships with others.

IV. Not occurring exclusively during the course of delirium.

 V. Either A or B:
   A. there is evidence from the history, physical examination, or laboratory tests of a specific organic factor (or factors) judged to be etiologically related to the disturbance
   B. in the absence of such evidence, an etiologic factor can be presumed if the disturbance cannot be accounted for by any nonorganic mental disorder, e.g., major depression accounting for cognitive impairment

VI. Insidious onset with a generally progressive deteriorating course.

VII. Exclusion of all other specific causes of dementia by history, physical examination, and laboratory tests.

Criteria for severity of Dementia:
   Mild: Although work or social activities are significantly impaired, the capacity for independent living remains, with adequate personal hygiene and relatively intact judgment.
   Moderate: Independent living is hazardous, and some degree of supervision is necessary.
   Severe: Activities of daily living are so impaired that continual supervision is required, e.g., unable to maintain personal hygiene; largely incoherent or mute.

Source: Reprinted with permission from the *Diagnostic and Statistical Manual of Mental Disorders, Third Edition, Revised.* Copyright 1987 American Psychiatric Association.

for both groups are similar (see also Jarvik, Chapter 13), the trend is not to differentiate between the senile and presenile forms. Although stages of Alzheimer's disease have been described (Reisberg, 1984; Berg, 1988), there is no firm scientific basis for precisely delineating these stages. The course of Alzheimer's disease is quite variable. Early in the disease, decreased energy, loss of interest in activities, lability of mood, and increased anxiety are common. The patient may be aware of these losses. Typically it begins with mild cognitive or personality changes and progresses with increasingly severe intellectual, social, and physical disability until eventually the patient becomes unable to carry out even the simplest activities of daily living. The configuration of the symptom complex may vary remarkably from patient to patient. Similarly, the tempo of the relentless decline varies considerably, with some patients enjoying years of relative stability. Stressful situations tend to precipitate symptoms.

Incontinence, gait disorders, and speech deterioration presage the terminal phase, during which the patient is often bedridden and unable to communicate verbally or nonverbally. The patient may vegetate until an infection, such as pneumonia or sepsis from a pressure sore, proves fatal. Most patients are thought to die within ten years of diagnosis.*

The physical examination, emphasizing neurologic function, may reveal other conditions whose signs and symptoms overlap with those of Alzheimer's disease, for example, Parkinson's disease and multiinfarct dementia (Hachinski et al., 1975). The mental-status examination should include evaluation of orientation, short- and long-term memory, recall, calculation, abstract thinking, judgment, and emotional state (Council on Scientific Affairs, 1986).

Since to date no single laboratory test is diagnostic of the disease, laboratory evaluation is aimed at identifying other treatable conditions that can mimic Alzheimer's disease. The Council on Scientific Affairs of the American Medical Association recommends the following measures: complete blood count; determination of electrolytes, serum glucose, serum urea nitrogen, and creatinine values; liver and thyroid function tests; serological test for syphilis; toxicology screen; determination of B_{12} and folate concentrations; sedimentation rate; urinalysis; chest roentgenogram; and electrocardiogram. If no abnormalities are found or if the abnormalities do not readily explain the patient's dementia, an electroen-

---

*Editors' Note: Older studies (Larson et al., 1963; Kay et al., 1964) noted a decreased life expectancy in patients with Alzheimer's disease, i.e., 2.3 to 2.6 years. However, patients previously came to the attention of medical professionals at a late stage of the disease. Because awareness of the disease is greater today, patients are seeking medical advice earlier, thereby enabling Alzheimer's disease to be diagnosed at a less advanced stage. Clinical experience documents that patients may live 20 years with the diagnosis. However, life expectancy data for Alzheimer patients is confounded by the difficulties in identifying both the onset of the disease and the cause of death, and death certificates are likely to underreport Alzheimer's disease in favor of cardiopulmonary arrest (Barclay et al., 1985).

cephalogram, a computed tomographic scan, and/or a lumbar puncture are recommended (Council on Scientific Affairs, 1986; U.S. Veteran's Administration, 1985).

The sensitivity and specificity of test-ordering strategies for patients with Alzheimer's disease have not been extensively studied, but Larson and his colleagues (1986) identified a Selective Test-Ordering Strategy. Their screening laboratory tests include complete blood count, chemistry battery (specifically glucose, sodium, other electrolytes, calcium, and creatinine), and thyrotropin (TSH) concentration. These authors offer guidelines for selective use of other tests, emphasizing that any strategy for test ordering should be employed with discretion and clinical judgment: (1) serum thyroxine (T_4) and triiodothyronine resin uptake (T_3RU) in patients with elevated concentrations of thyrotropin; (2) serum cyanocobalamin and serum or red blood cell folate levels in patients with anemia and/or macrocytosis; and (3) repeated sodium, calcium, and glucose determinations if abnormal initially.

Computed tomographic (CT) brain scans are performed in clinical practice to rule out the possibilities of other diseases causing dementia, such as tumors or multiinfarct dementia (LeMay, 1986). Atrophy on a CT scan has a stronger correlation with advancing age than with dementia (Yerby et al., 1985). Based on review of 500 consecutive patients presenting for CT scans in Bristol, England, Bradshaw and his colleagues (1983) suggested that CT scans be performed on patients with specific diagnostic pointers (headache, focal signs, papilledema, and speech disorders) and on patients who have been demented for less than one year. Larson and his colleagues suggest that the CT scan is probably most useful for patients with recent onset of dementia or acute deterioration and in those with unexplained or atypical neurologic findings (Larson et al., 1986). More data are needed to determine the general applicability of these findings to other patient populations.

For research purposes, however, more stringent diagnostic procedures are needed to assure that subjects included do not have either coexistent illness or other causes of dementia. Guidelines for research purposes have been developed (McKhann et al., 1984).

Despite stringent clinical or research protocols, at the present time the diagnosis of Alzheimer's disease can only be made with certainty by autopsy or biopsy study of the brain. Pathologic alterations in the brain include senile plaque formation and neurofibrillary tangles to a degree not found in the normal aging process. Some patients who receive a diagnosis of Alzheimer's may be found to have other dementing illnesses at postmortem evaluation. Because autopsies validate the clinical diagnosis, they are often helpful to family members.

The unrelenting downward spiral of Alzheimer's disease frequently leads to a sense of pessimism and therapeutic nihilism among physicians and other health care professionals. But despite lack of medications to reverse the underlying etiology, physicians need not feel helpless or hopeless, because management strategies do exist that can help treat the manifestations of this disease (Winograd & Jarvik, 1986). Incurable does not mean untreatable. As with other chronic diseases, such as diabetes mellitus, congestive heart failure, or degenerative arthritis, curative remedies for the underlying disorder do not exist. Treatment is often symptomatic rather than pathology-specific. Similarly, with Alzheimer's disease we can develop a multipronged approach that will help preserve the patient's remaining abilities (Council on Scientific Affairs, 1986). Physicians need to develop management strategies that will: (1) treat the manifestations of Alzheimer's disease; (2) identify and treat coexistent illnesses; (3) institute periodic clinical review; (4) use a minimum of medications at nontoxic doses; (5) treat specific associated syndromes (e.g., nighttime wakening and fecal incontinence); and (6) provide support to caregivers.

TREATMENT OF MANIFESTATIONS OF ALZHEIMER'S DISEASE

Patients with Alzheimer's disease present with a variety of symptoms that physicians are asked to treat. Depending on the stage of disease, these include mild personality changes, day/night reversal, apathy, hostility, falls, wandering, and incontinence. When evaluating symptoms, clinicians need to consider whether they are more amenable to behavioral or to drug therapy. Changes in personality (e.g., the patient becomes more irritable) tend to be resistant to drug therapy but respond to behavioral treatments. Approaches that decrease confrontation often minimize the manifestations of these personality changes. Regular routines without surprise help Alzheimer patients stay calm, so that their functional abilities are maintained as much as possible. Table 1.2 provides suggestions that can enable patients to use their remaining abilities appropriately (see also Burnside, Chapter 2).

Some symptoms have proven responsive to appropriate drug therapy. For example, paranoid or hostile behavior may decrease with introduction of 0.5 mg of haloperidol once or twice a day as a starting dosage, with increases of 0.5 mg every three to four days if needed. Low dosages of haloperidol are unlikely to improve wandering, a use to which it has sometimes been put. The clinical adage of "start low, go slow" is especially appropriate for patients with drug-treatable syndromes. The corollary, "don't increase when the symptoms get better," should also be

TABLE 1.2 Environmental Support for Alzheimer Patient

I. Create a Stable, Dependable Setting
   A. Regular schedules
   B. Patient's possessions kept in same place
   C. Sequential locks on doors to prevent wandering
II. Minimize Confusion
   A. Provide as much environmental stimulation as patient can tolerate
   B. When patient begins to fidget or become tense from too much stimulation, reduce the following:
      1. activities
      2. conversations
      3. requests
      4. distractions
      5. number of visitors
      6. television
III. Provide and Enhance Multiple Sensory Cues
   A. Hearing-aid batteries maintained
   B. Glasses and dentures properly in place
   C. Lighting levels increased
   D. Night lights used
   E. Clocks available
IV. Reassess Patient's Safety Regularly
   A. Review patient's capacity for independent function
      1. cooking
      2. smoking
      3. living alone
      4. risk of falling
   B. Assess environment for potential hazardous situations
      1. unstable furniture and rugs
      2. stairs
      3. matches and/or gas stoves
      4. bathrooms
      5. electric wiring
V. Communicate with Concise and Simple Statements
   A. Provide one-step units of information and/or instructions
   B. Use only positive information, when possible
   C. Avoid negative commands, such as "don't do that," that confuse the patient
   D. Use distractions as a response to perseveration and undesirable behavior
      1. motor distraction is more effective than verbal requests
      2. if patient is pulling caregiver's hair, ask the patient to hold something else; this is more effective than telling patient to stop
VI. Learning Routines
   A. Schedule demanding tasks for the patient's best time of day
   B. Readjust tasks frequently to fit the patient's level of functions
      1. assign tasks that the patient is capable of performing so that the patient maintains some control over his/her environment
      2. change expectations when inability to perform a previously easy task occurs

Source: Adapted from Council on Scientific Affairs (1986). Used with permission.

followed. Once improvement has been attained, increased dosages are unlikely to result in further clinical improvement and may cause adverse side effects.

In patients with mild to moderate dementia, ergoloid mesylates (1–2 mg three times a day for 3–6 months) may help improve mobility or self-care but usually do not produce meaningful improvement of cognitive function (Hollister & Yesavage, 1984). For patients with depressive symptomatology, a trial of antidepressants or psychotherapy is warranted. The initial choice of therapy depends on the symptom complex. Agitated patients with insomnia may do best with a sedating drug such as trazodone or doxepin. For most other patients, desipramine may be more appropriate because it has relatively fewer anticholinergic and orthostatic side effects (see also Satlin & Cole, Chapter 3).

TREATMENT OF COEXISTENT ILLNESS

The prevalence of depression in patients with Alzheimer's disease has been reported by Reifler and his colleagues. In their study of 88 cognitively impaired geriatric outpatients, patients with mild dementia (33%), moderate dementia (28%), and severe dementia (12%) also suffered from depressive illness (Reifler et al., 1982). The recognition of this affective disorder is important because it is amenable to psychotherapy, behavioral, and/or pharmacologic therapy (see also Cohen, Chapter 5; Tune et al., Chapter 7; Reifler et al., 1986; Winograd & Jarvik, 1986).

The prevalence of coexistent delirium in community-dwelling patients with Alzheimer's disease has not been studied, but a major British study documented that approximately one-third of hospitalized patients with dementia had a superimposed delirium (College Committee on Geriatrics, 1981). A high index of suspicion for this treatable condition is essential to diagnose the underlying medical conditions that cause it (Lipowski, 1983).

Other medical conditions may also coexist with Alzheimer's disease. Diseases that are common among the aged, such as diabetes mellitus and coronary artery disease, are thought to be less prevalent in patients with Alzheimer's disease than in the general population, but the true prevalence is unknown. Many patients undergoing evaluation for Alzheimer's disease are found to have more than one illness contributing to the dementia state.

Larson and his colleagues identified medical diseases in over 50% of patients undergoing comprehensive diagnostic evaluation for suspected dementia. The authors observed that over 30% of patients had more than one condition contributing to the dementia state. The most common new diagnoses of so-called treatable illnesses were drug toxicity, hypothyroidism, low serum folate, osteoarthritis, Parkinson's disease, and urinary tract infection. Improvement occurred in nearly 30% of patients and persisted in 14% for at least one year. However, only two patients out of 200 recovered normal mental function (Larson et al., 1985).

Not only is the actual prevalence of medical conditions unknown, but data are also lacking about their specific impact on demented patients. Medical conditions not generally thought to cause central nervous system (CNS) impairment may affect cognitive function in these patients because their reserve mental capacity is so limited that any illness may further compromise cognitive function. Effective therapy of conditions such as congestive heart failure, chronic obstructive pulmonary disease, and constipation may lead to both functional and cognitive improvements.

Any acute or subacute change that occurs over time may point to intercurrent illness. For example, recent onset of incontinence, new onset of wandering, or the emergence of violent behavior may herald underlying medical illnesses. When Alzheimer patients experience myocardial infarction or pneumonia, deterioration in cognitive function may be the presenting symptom. Data do not exist at present to help clinicians differentiate the deterioration due to intercurrent illness from that of the disease process itself. A careful medical evaluation should be performed whenever an acute or subacute deterioration occurs in either cognitive or behavioral function. Intercurrent illnesses are frequently treatable, and appropriate therapy may allow patients to return to their previous level of function. Unfortunately, despite therapy some patients remain at a lower level of function. No clinical indicators are currently known to help clinicians predict which patients are likely to improve.

The impact of comorbid conditions on the progression of Alzheimer's disease has not been well documented, but preliminary studies suggest that their presence may cause excess disability (see also Cohen, Chapter 5). Uhlmann and colleagues have studied the relationship of hearing loss to cognitive function, correlating the finger friction test (e.g., ability to hear fingers being rubbed together at the ear) with the Mini-Mental State (Folstein et al., 1975). They found that over a one-year follow-up period, those patients who could not hear the finger friction test had a greater decline in the Mini-Mental State than those whose hearing was intact. Although the clinical significance of this statistically significant decline is not known, it suggests that sensory impairment may contribute to excess morbidity in demented patients (Uhlmann et al., 1986).

Buchner and Larson, studying falls in demented patients, found that those who fell tended to have reversible dementias, caused primarily by drug toxicity. Fallers also suffered frequently from arthritis and Parkinson's disease, which are amenable to therapy. Thus falls may be a marker for medication toxicity, may be preventable, or may be a sentinel event suggesting some other underlying illness (Buchner & Larson, 1986).

INSTITUTION OF PERIODIC REVIEW

Patients with Alzheimer's disease exhibit substantial changes in their clinical and social condition over time. To identify problems such as impaired mobility, loss of self-care capacity, financial burden, or caregiver stress, physicians need to assess patients at specific intervals. When the course of the disease is relatively stable, evaluation every three to six months in a multidisciplinary clinic with telephone follow-up by a nurse or social worker between visits provides adequate clinical information to treat incipient conditions. In primary-care settings (e.g., doctors' offices), shorter, more frequent visits are also effective. These planned visits help avoid overburdening the family or patient with excessive medical care and can help minimize clinical crises (see also Tune et al., Chapter 7).

When diagnosis and treatment are based at a tertiary-care center (e.g., university hospital referral center), it is often helpful for the patient also to have a primary-care physician (an internist, family practitioner, or psychiatrist) involved in the ongoing care. Communication between the primary physician and the referral center is essential for coordinated care (Council on Scientific Affairs, 1986).

Periodic evaluation should include assessment of medical and psychiatric conditions, including review of medications. Care needs and functional status of the patient should be reviewed, along with social supports and caregiver needs. Table 1.3 lists four areas to be addressed in the course of ongoing care, with specific items to address in each category. All professionals caring for the patient can participate in the process of gathering these data. Not all areas need to be addressed at every visit, but over the course of a year, assessment of each of these areas should occur.

Evaluation of needs should be followed by a family discussion of plans to handle events expected in the next three to six months. Health care providers can assist families in this process by providing stage-appropriate anticipatory guidance. For example, in the early stages, the patient and family would be alerted to issues likely to come up about continued employment. Early discussion of feelings about nursing homes

TABLE 1.3 Periodic Review: Checklist for Patients with Dementia

I. Medical and Psychiatric Condition
   A. Medications
   B. Coexistent medical illnesses
   C. Nutrition
   D. Anorexia
   E. Sleep disturbance
   F. Neurological changes
   G. Incontinence
   H. Sexual problems, disinhibitions
   I. Depression
   J. Agitated, restless, irritable behavior
   K. Inappropriate affect
   L. Suspicious, paranoid thoughts
   M. Hostility, verbal and physical threats
   N. Dental conditions
   O. Foot problems
II. Care Needs of Patient
   A. Activity and functional status
      1. what is patient's daily schedule?
      2. does patient wander? get lost?
      3. activities of daily living (see Appendix 3)
      4. instrumental activities of daily living (see Appendix 5)
      5. does patient drive? problems?
      6. does patient use or abuse drugs or alcohol?
      7. who supervises medications?
      8. who handles finances?
   B. Social skills
      1. what are patient's social activities?
      2. with whom does patient have relationships?
      3. how does patient react to visitors?
      4. how does patient react to change in environment (e.g., likes or panics in restaurant)
III. Social Supports
   A. Living arrangements
      1. housing
      2. financial resources
   B. Human resources
      1. available family
      2. available friends
      3. counseling
      4. in-home services
IV. Caregiver Needs
   A. Social supports
      1. respite services
      2. support group
      3. financial aid
      4. available friends and family

(*continued*)

TABLE 1.3 *(continued)*

    B. Psychological issues
        1. evidence of depression
        2. evidence of other psychopathology
        3. abuse by patient
        4. abuse of patient
    C. Medical issues
        1. symptoms of physical illness?
        2. use of drugs? alcohol?
        3. sleep disturbance?
        4. health habits?
    D. Legal
        1. property
        2. durable power of attorney
        3. arrangements for decisions regarding medical treatment; durable power of attorney for health, living will

---

and, when appropriate, visits to facilities under consideration might be encouraged. In late stages, questions would be asked about planning for treatment of acute medical illness, including use of ventilators and nasogastric tubes. Periodic family conferences can help patients and caregivers maintain sufficient confidence to handle a changing and difficult situation (see also Tune et al., Chapter 7).

Where multidisciplinary teams are available, health professionals from different disciplines can address specific aspects to help facilitate efficiency in caring for these patients. Social workers can assess social supports; nurses, functional status; and physicians, medications and incontinence. However, because the care of these patients requires coordination among many disciplines, all professionals working with these patients need to have broad-based knowledge of patients, families, and the disease itself. For example, physicians need to know about functional status and support systems in order to evaluate appropriately symptoms of psychopathology.

To help identify cognitive and functional abilities, we recommend administering one or more of the following brief screening instruments: the Mini-Mental State Examination (Folstein et al., 1975); Clinical Dementia Rating (CDR) Scale (Berg, 1988); Index of Independence in Activities of Daily Living (Katz et al., 1970); Physical Self-Maintenance Scale (Lawton & Brody, 1969); and Instrumental Activities of Daily Living (Lawton et al., 1982) (see Appendices 1, 2, 3, 4, and 5, respectively). For patients clinically considered to have coexistent depression, the Geriatric Depression Scale (Short Form) (Sheikh & Yesavage, 1986), the Hamilton Rating Scale for Depression (Hamilton, 1960), and the

Zung Self-Rating Depression Scale (Zung, 1965) (see Appendices 6, 7, and 8) may also be helpful. We cannot stress enough that *regardless of the severity of dementia, no rating scale by itself can make the diagnosis* of either dementia or depression, just as no laboratory test by itself can diagnose a medical condition.

Another reason for periodic review of Alzheimer patients is that despite a thorough and appropriate initial investigation, the diagnosis may be in error. Indeed, studies of patients thought to have presenile dementia have documented an incidence of erroneous diagnosis as high as 57% (Ron et al., 1979; Nott & Fleminger, 1975). Severe neurotic or affective disorders commonly were misdiagnosed as dementia. Patients may improve over time either through the benefit of treatment of coexistent illnesses or through the "tincture of time."

The problem of false positive diagnosis has not been studied adequately among patients in their seventies and eighties. Clinical lore suggests that false positive diagnoses occur in approximately 10% to 20% of cases in this age group, and some research documents this (Sulkava et al., 1983). The clinical caveat remains: Alzheimer's disease cannot yet be definitively diagnosed without an autopsy. When diagnosis is uncertain, it is preferable to err on the side of *not* labeling the patient as demented. When patients have been so labeled yet improve in their cognitive and behavioral function, we recommend formal neuropsychological testing. If the results of this testing show the patient to be completely normal, then the diagnosis of dementia can be eliminated from their record. When some improvement occurs but cognitive impairment still exists, we caution the patient and caregiver that only with time will we have a better understanding of the condition. When the progression of disease is atypical, further medical or psychiatric evaluation or neuropsychological testing is indicated to document the specific cognitive losses and identify potentially treatable etiologies.

Periodic review can also benefit caregivers, enabling them to identify areas of concern so that specific interventions can occur. We have found in clinical practice that unless we specifically question caregivers about incontinence, they are unlikely to volunteer the information. Amazingly, many caregivers cope with makeshift diaper arrangements and are reluctant to ask for professional assistance. Identification of problems with self-care may lead to referral for in-home or respite services. Social isolation should prompt referral to a caregiver support group (Barnes et al., 1981) such as those sponsored by the Alzheimer's Disease and Related Disorders Association (ADRDA) (see also Brody, Chapter 6; Tune et al., Chapter 7; Reveley, Chapter 8; Sainer, Chapter 11).

MEDICATION STRATEGY

Elderly people seem to be more sensitive than middle-aged people to the adverse effects of pharmacologic agents (Jarvik et al., 1981). Many experienced clinicians believe that demented patients may be more sensitive to drugs than nondemented adults, especially to psychotropics and analgesics. Adverse drug reactions are an important source of excess disability in patients with dementia or suspected dementia. Larson and his associates recently documented how the use of sedative hypnotics and antihypertensives is strongly associated with cognitive impairment due to adverse drug reactions (Larson et al., 1987). When reviewing medications, it is best to consider that almost any drug may cause cognitive impairment. Table 1.4 lists some of the major drugs that can cause adverse effects in the central nervous system (CNS). Some drugs produce these effects as part of their mechanism of action (e.g., barbiturates or benzodiazepines). More troublesome are those drugs that cause CNS effects unpredictably, such as glucocorticoids or nonsteroidal antiinflammatory agents, and that are used for frequently severe and debilitating conditions. Nearly 100 drugs have been reported to cause psychiatric symptoms. These reports are limited to single drugs in all ages. Drug interactions may also cause adverse psychiatric reactions ("Drugs that Cause Psychiatric Symptoms," 1986). Clinicians should be alert to drugs, including over-the-counter remedies, that are generally

---

TABLE 1.4 Drugs Causing Central Nervous System (CNS) Effects

  I. Unpredictable CNS Effects
    A. Glucocorticoids (steroids)
    B. Nonsteroidal antiinflammatory agents
    C. H_2 blockers (Cimetidine, Ranitidine)
    D. Antihistamines
    E. Decongestants
  II. Predictable CNS Effects
    A. Phenothiazines
    B. Barbiturates
    C. Benzodiazepines
 III. Metabolic Toxicities
    A. Insulin
    B. Sulfonylureas
    C. Diuretics
 IV. Taken Incorrectly
    A. Digoxin
    B. Aspirin

---

innocuous in younger patients but may cause adverse side effects in the elderly. We have seen patients on small doses of decongestant-antihistamines whose cognitive function improved substantially when these medications were discontinued.

Eliminating as many medications as possible without causing exacerbation of other illnesses is the desired goal. Often patients can safely undergo a nondrug trial during which the severity of the underlying clinical conditions can be evaluated. Two different approaches are recommended, depending on the severity of the situation and the clinical resources. The first approach is elimination, one by one, of drugs known to cause CNS side effects (such as sedative hypnotics), leaving other drugs as originally prescribed. If no improvement occurs, remaining drugs, if not essential, are removed sequentially. The order of elimination is determined by balancing the frequency of CNS side effects against efficacy for other conditions and the patient's presumed need. When patients are on multiple medications, this approach may take considerable time before a baseline cognitive state is achieved.

The second approach is more radical but often effective. All drugs that can be safely discontinued are stopped and the rest are tapered. The patient is monitored closely to identify the severity of underlying conditions and to establish a nondrug baseline of cognitive functioning. Should an exacerbation of the patient's medical illnesses occur, for example, deterioration of congestive heart failure or severe pain, necessary drugs can be instituted at the lowest possible dosages and titrated upward as indicated. If possible, monitoring the patient several times weekly at home is preferable to office visits or hospitalization. Because of the long half-lives of many drugs (e.g., benzodiazepines and digoxin) in the elderly, several weeks may elapse before the true baseline is achieved. Hospitalizing the patient does facilitate monitoring, but it may cause increased confusion due to environmental stress and related iatrogenic conditions (Steel, 1984). Moreover, prolonged hospitalization is frequently not economically feasible. Research data are unavailable, but geriatricians have found that some "demented" patients can be "cured" by discontinuing medications.

TREATMENT OF SPECIFIC SYNDROMES

The Alzheimer patient is beset with a variety of clinical conditions that are amenable to medical intervention (Winograd & Jarvik, 1986). The focus of this section is on two conditions: nighttime wakening and fecal incontinence. These conditions deserve close attention not only because they are common in Alzheimer patients, but also because they are amenable to therapy. Moreover, they present substantial challenges to caregivers and often precipitate institutionalization. Fecal incontinence, in particular, requires detailed exposition, since its physiology and treatment are not widely understood.

Sanford (1975) studied long-term caregivers of recently institutionalized patients. He asked which problems would have to be alleviated to allow the patient to return home. He found that sleep disturbances, including night wandering, incontinence, and shouting, were the behaviors that led most frequently to institutionalization. Although fecal incontinence was less common than urinary incontinence, caregivers were less tolerant of this condition. Fecal incontinence was more likely to contribute to institutionalization than was urinary incontinence.

Nighttime Wakening

Sleep changes occur with aging. The normal elderly have more awakenings, more Stage 1 (early, light sleep) and less Stages 3 and 4 (deep) sleep than young or middle-aged adults (Miles & Dement, 1980). Patients with mild dementia living in the community show even less Stages 3 and 4 sleep and more frequent awakenings (Prinz et al., 1982a) than normal elderly. Patients with moderate or severe dementia also show decreased rapid-eye-movement (REM) time and increased REM latency (Vitiello et al., 1984; Prinz et al., 1982b). The impaired sleep, observed even in early Alzheimer's disease, and the night wandering may be related to each other and to the underlying pathophysiology of the disease itself. Thus Prinz hypothesizes that neuronal degeneration in the sleep-regulation center (locus ceruleus) may be etiologically related to fragmentation of the sleep–wake pattern (Prinz et al., 1982a, 1982b). Although controversy exists about the crucial regulatory pathways that underlie the sleep changes noted in Alzheimer patients, a striking similarity has been noted between the distribution of neurofibrillary tangles in Alzheimer's disease and the neuronal pathways thought to be responsible for both REM and non-REM sleep (Rossi, 1972; Ishii, 1966).

In addition to impairment of sleep caused by pathophysiologic changes, demented patients are also at risk for other causes of sleep disturbance that affect older patients. Controversy exists about the role of myoclonus (shocklike contractions of a portion of a muscle, or a group of muscles, restricted to one area of the body or appearing synchronously or asynchronously in several places) and sleep apnea (transient attacks of failure of automatic control of respiration, resulting in alveolar hypoventilation, which becomes pronounced during sleep) in geriatric insomnia. Some sleep laboratories have documented a high frequency of these disorders among insomniacs (Roehrs et al., 1985; Coleman et al., 1981; Roehrs et al., 1983). Others reported equal prevalence in individuals with and without complaints of insomnia (Bliwise et al., 1987; Kales et al., 1982). For Alzheimer patients the evidence is mixed, but overall there seems to be rough equivalence with elderly controls (Reynolds et al., 1985; Bliwise et al., 1986; Frommlet et al., 1986; Prinz et al., 1986; Smallwood et al., 1983). Drugs, such as some antihypertensives (e.g., beta blockers), corticosteroids, antiarrhythmics, and anti-parkinsonians, can produce nightmares and nighttime awakenings (Guilleminault & Silvestri, 1982). Decreasing dosage and discontinuing medication, when possible, may improve sleep.

Clinically, we find that hunger may cause impaired sleep and bedtime snacks may improve sleeping (Southwell et al., 1972). Anecdotal experience suggests that one-third to one-half of patients who snack seem to sleep better. At least caregivers report that sleep problems are relieved. Care must be taken not to induce weight gain with the nighttime snack, because increased sleep apnea has been associated with weight gains of 10 to 20 pounds (Bliwise et al., 1984). Similarly, in obese subjects moderate weight loss can decrease sleep apnea, improve sleep pattern, and decrease daytime hypersomnolence (Smith PL et al., 1985).

Other common causes of insomnia, especially in hospital and institutional settings, include pain, night cramps in legs, nocturia, fear, and environmental disruption (Berlin, 1984). These conditions need investigation and appropriate treatment. When patients have nocturia because they are taking diuretics at night, the drugs can be taken in the morning. Clinical experience supports treating patients with leg cramps with foot boards, quinine (Gootnick, 1943), exercises (Weiner & Weiner, 1980), diphenhydramine (50 mg), and/or vitamin E (Ayres & Mihan, 1974).

Fear and decreased sensory input may be important factors in inducing nighttime wandering, agitation, and the poorly understood phenomenon of "sundowning." Cameron's old study (1941) of patients suffering from nocturnal delirium suggests that patients develop delirium when deprived of visual cues because of severe impairment in their capacity to retain what they saw. Unable to maintain a spatial image without the assistance of repeated visualizations, these patients cannot locate themselves in space during the night and, therefore, feel insecure and anxious. Perhaps this explains why use of nightlights and attention to appropriate environmental stimuli (e.g., familiar photographs, decorations, soothing colors) can reduce "sundowning" and decrease nighttime wandering and agitation (see also Burnside, Chapter 2).

Even after treating underlying and exacerbating causes of insomnia, many demented patients still exhibit impaired sleep. Unfortunately, systematic studies on treatment of sleep disturbance in Alzheimer's disease do not exist, but clinicians have developed various treatment strategies. When insomnia is not stressful to the patient and when the patient's awakenings do not interfere with the caregivers' sleep, no therapy is necessary. However, the patient often sleeps for only short intervals at a time, and the caregiver, not being prepared for this, has his or her own sleep impaired. This may result in fatigue, anxiety, depression, or medical illness for the caregiver. Thus a major problem with nighttime wakening is its deleterious effect on caregivers. Explaining to caregivers the nature of the sleep disturbance and helping them create a safe environment (e.g., use of low beds if mobility permits so that patients cannot injure themselves) may help relieve caregiver anxiety. Caregivers may also be concerned that the abnormal sleep may be detrimental to the patient's condition. Since we have no data about the long-term effect of impaired sleep on cognitive function, we should be careful not to give false assurances. However, we need to explain to caregivers that depriving themselves of sleep serves neither the patient nor anyone else.

For most patients, behavioral management strategies can improve sleep (Table 1.5) (see also Burnside, Chapter 2). Clinical experience suggests that physical exercise may improve sleep, and some sleep laboratory studies in younger individuals support this clinical finding (Horne, 1981). Daytime activities such as walking, gardening, or playing ball might improve nighttime sleep while maintaining physical conditioning. Alzheimer patients frequently doze on and off all day long. Clinical experience suggests that minimizing naps or avoiding them completely often improves nighttime sleep, though data are available only for non-

---

TABLE 1.5 Management of Insomnia in the Demented Patient

- Ascertain and treat underlying etiology (e.g., pain, fear, drug side effects)
- Try to avoid nighttime fluids and diuretics
- Treat painful conditions (e.g., nocturnal leg muscle cramps)
- Try to minimize fear and disorientation
- Encourage moderate physical exercise during the day (e.g., walking, swimming)
- Try to keep patient dressed during usual waking hours
- Try to minimize naps, but do not deprive patient of needed rest
- Consider bedtime snacks
- Consider use of warm milk (4–8 oz) and tryptophan (1500 mg), when patients are milk intolerant, warm decaffeinated or herbal tea can be substituted
- Consider warm bath prior to sleep
- For discussion of drugs, see text

---

demented subjects (Spielman et al., 1983; Saskin et al., 1984). Daytime wakefulness may be facilitated by having patients dressed and out of bed. Keeping the bedrails up during the day may deter afternoon napping by making it difficult for hospitalized or institutionalized patients to lie down. However, restraints and bedrails at night should be used rarely, if at all. They frequently cause agitation in demented patients and may not protect them from falling. Restrained patients may fall from a greater height, thereby increasing the probability of serious injury. Whenever possible, putting the mattress close to the floor is a safe alternative for the demented patient who gets out of bed at night. Care must be taken to assure that frail patients are able to raise themselves from the low bed.

When behavioral-management techniques are insufficient to resolve the sleep problem, additional therapy may be indicated. Our first choice is a warm nighttime beverage. Investigators have shown improved sleep with hot milk drinks (Southwell et al., 1972; Brezinova & Oswald, 1972). Many patients report that warm milk or tea (preferably herbal or decaffeinated) at bedtime helps them sleep. If this is ineffective, tryptophan (1500 mg) can be started. Circulating plasma L-tryptophan levels increase brain serotonin levels, and exogenous administration of L-tryptophan (1–4 gm) has been shown to decrease waking time and sleep latency (time needed to fall asleep) (Hartmann, 1977; Spinweber et al., 1983), although these effects may take more than one week to occur (Hartmann et al., 1983). Although not specifically studied in demented patients, L-tryptophan at low doses is safe with minimal side effects (Pakes, 1979). The data are scanty and controversial, but some investigators have raised the question of an association of tryptophan metabolites in bladder and breast cancer (Dunning et al., 1950; Rose & Randall, 1973), while other investigators disagree (Price, 1966). Further work is needed to elucidate what role dietary tryptophan may have on carcinogenesis. Tryptophan is often effective for mild to moderate sleep disturbances for about three months, at which time its effectiveness seems to wear off. Improvement in the patient's sleep, although temporary, frequently helps caregivers get some sleep themselves.

When L-tryptophan is not effective, chloral hydrate (0.5 gm) may be a reasonable choice because of its short half-life (8–11 hours) and low frequency of side effects. In one study CNS side effects of depression or excitation occurred in only 1% of hospitalized patients, less than with other sedative hypnotic drugs. Patients at risk for adverse reactions were those over age 50 who were severely ill, who were concurrently receiving benzodiazepines, and who had elevated blood urea nitrogen levels. Sensitivity reactions and gastrointestinal disturbances were even less frequent. Its efficacy was comparable to the other hypnotics used for hospitalized patients in this study (Miller RR & Greenblatt, 1979). Data for demented elderly patients could not be found in the literature. The effectiveness of chloral hydrate may wear off after 10 days, but the situation for the caregiver may improve with 10 days of sleep. Withdrawal of chloral hydrate may be associated with insomnia (Linnoila et al., 1980).

The very short-acting (e.g., triazolam, half-life 1.5–5.0 hours) and intermediate-acting (e.g., temazepam, half-life 8–38 hours) benzodiazepines produce fewer side effects than do the long-acting ones. Data on demented elderly are scanty (see also Satlin and Cole, Chapter 3). In geriatric insomniacs, triazolam 0.25 mg has decreased sleep latency, increased sleep duration, and decreased the number of nocturnal awakenings (Okawa, 1978; Reeves, 1977). Sleep electroencephalogram studies have shown no effect on sleep Stages 3 and 4 and variable effects on REM sleep. The most common side effects are similar to those of other benzodiazepines, including residual drowsiness, headache, dizziness, nervousness, and dry mouth; but Pakes and colleagues (1981) reported that the incidence of these side effects with 0.25 mg of triazolam was generally no greater than after placebo. Upon withdrawal of triazolam, sleep parameters (i.e., sleep latency, total sleep time, and number of awakenings) generally approach baseline levels but do not exceed them (Kroboth & Juhl, 1983). We recommend an initial dose of 0.125 mg in demented patients, which can be increased up to 0.25 mg at bedtime with careful monitoring of side effects.

Because temazepam has a delayed peak effect (up to three hours), it must be given two hours before bedtime. Doses of 15 to 30 mg increase total sleep time and decrease nocturnal awakenings but do not decrease sleep latency. Temazepam redistributes REM sleep and decreases sleep Stages 3 and 4. It can produce confusion, dizziness, and drowsiness in elderly patients. Accumulation and concomitant morning hangover may occur with repeated use (Wincor, 1982).

For depressed, demented patients with sleep disturbance, doxepin (25 to 50 mg) is a reasonable choice because of its sedative action. Trazodone (50 to 100 mg) can also be used for its sedative action. Although free from anticholinergic side effects, it has not yet been widely used for Alzheimer patients. Its alpha-adrenergic properties sometimes cause dry mouth and blurred vision, which may be thought to indicate anticholinergic side effects. For agitated, paranoid patients, thioridazine (15 to 25 mg) can be considered. However, its anticholinergic properties may exacerbate cognitive impairment (see also Satlin and Cole, Chapter 3).

Both environmental and drug therapies have their limitations. Once nighttime wandering becomes a problem it tends to persist and cause caregiver stress. Environmental manipulations facilitate more sleep during nighttime hours. However, vigilance over these interventions is needed to maintain their effectiveness. Drug therapies, although frequently helpful initially, eventually lose their effectiveness as patients become tolerant to the drugs. Consequently, it makes sense to institute one intervention at a time to maximize its therapeutic value. When no longer effective, another therapy, either environmental or pharmacological, can be instituted. We recommend planning for serial therapies, either pharmacological or nonpharmacological, realizing that the effects of most interventions last only weeks to months.

Fecal Incontinence

Fecal incontinence is the inability to control the excrement (stool) discharged from the intestines. The prevalence of fecal incontinence among Alzheimer patients is unknown. Published data from the United Kingdom suggest rates of 10% to 23% (Brocklehurst, 1951; Wilkin & Jolley, 1978; Dodd et al., 1979) among patients in long-stay wards and residential homes, but this may represent underreporting. Smith reports his own data on 112 patients in a geriatric unit who were followed carefully by a research nurse; 53% were incontinent of feces occasionally (at least once per week) and 14% had persistent incontinence (more than three times per week). Fecal smearing, which is often not considered incontinence by nursing staff, accounted for 41% of the episodes. Smith noted that persistently incontinent patients in his study were demented, very demanding, or both, and were unpopular with the staff (Smith RG, 1983). These data support clinical experience that severely demented patients frequently have fecal incontinence and present a substantial burden to caregivers.

Pathophysiology

Research on the anatomy and physiology of continence is fraught with controversy over techniques, results, and small numbers of subjects (Dickinson, 1978). The discussion that follows attempts to present a consensus of existing scientific literature and is divided into two sections: (1) fecal impaction, resulting in fecal soiling and (2) impairment of mechanisms that maintain continence.

Fecal Impaction The most common cause of fecal soiling in Alzheimer patients is commonly termed "overflow incontinence." This condition, which is not truly an impairment of the continence mechanism, is caused by fecal impaction, which is the end result of conditions causing constipation (Table 1.6). Increased transit time leads to progressive fecal stasis, constipation, and finally impaction. This decreased gastrointestinal motility results from several factors, including diet lacking in fiber, inactivity, changes in gastrointestinal hormones, neuronal damages, and, perhaps, aging per se.

Severely prolonged transit time with impaction leads to fecal soiling. The consistency of the leaked feces can be hard, soft, or liquid and may be mistaken for diarrhea. Two patterns of impaction occur. The first type is colonic, with prolonged transit time throughout the entire colon. Water absorption is increased, producing small, hard feces. The second type, dyschezic impaction, has a normal transit time through the descending and transverse colon, so that water absorption is normal. Movement is delayed through the sigmoid to the rectum, producing distention of the left side of the colon with a large amount of soft feces. Persistent distention of the rectum with a large bolus of feces will lead to passage of liquid or soft stool around the impacted mass (Parks, 1980; Smith RG, 1983). Leakage of stool may occur even when the neuromuscular mechanisms to maintain continence remain intact. When the constipated state is chronic, the rectum becomes distended, the sphincters lose tone, and the anus becomes patulous. Clinically, stool leaks frequently, soils clothing without relation to meals, and leads to substantial caregiver burden.

TABLE 1.6 Causes of Constipation

I. Fecal Stasis
    A. Decreased fiber
    B. Decreased fluids
    C. Decreased exercise
    D. Bedrest
II. Medications
    A. Anticholinergics
    B. Narcotics
    C. Iron
    D. Diuretics
    E. Aluminum-containing antacids
III. Carcinoma
IV. Neurologic Disorders
    A. Cortical (e.g., Alzheimer's disease)
    B. Spinal (e.g., compressive syndromes)
    C. Peripheral neuropathy (e.g., diabetes mellitus)

Mechanisms to Maintain Fecal Continence To control defecation, continence requires the ability both to discriminate between solid, liquid, and gas in the anorectal region and to defer excretory function to a convenient time and place (Peck, 1980). The anal sphincter mechanism is a wonder of anatomy and physiology. The nerve endings that line the anal canal (i.e., part of the anoderm) differentiate gas from solid or liquid (Duthie & Gairns, 1960). Figure 1.1 shows a schematic diagram of the anatomy of continence. The anal canal is approximately 4 cm long. The anorectal junction is maintained at a right angle by the levator ani muscle, a wide curved sheet of muscle that forms the pelvic floor. The puborectalis, a major part of the levator ani, serves as a sling for the lower rectum and anal canal. The proximal (upper) part of the anal canal is flattened and closed by the weight of the abdominal organs pushing down on the anterior wall of the rectum. This creates a flap valve mechanism, which helps prevent fecal seepage into the anus. Any increase in intra-abdominal pressure increases this valve effect by compressing the lower rectal wall more firmly on the closed upper anal canal (Sullivan ES et al., 1982).

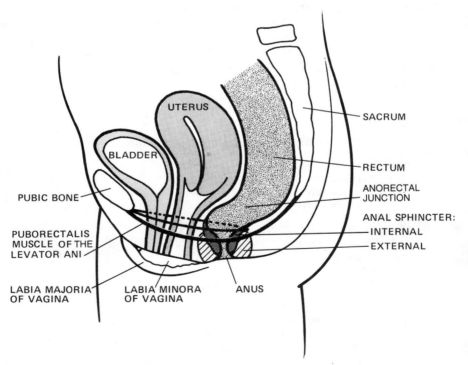

FIGURE 1.1 Pelvic anatomy: lateral view (see text for further details).

Continence is maintained by a complex of visceral and somatic factors. The visceral (or involuntary) factors located in the rectum and the anal canal are innervated by the autonomic nervous system.

Somatic (or voluntary) factors act on the external sphincter muscles and the puborectalis of levator ani via a spinal reflex arc (Figure 1.2). The deep portion of the external sphincter combines with the puborectalis of the levator ani muscle, which fans out via the iliococcygeus and pubococcygeus muscles to prevent herniation of the rectum and lower bowel (Parks, 1980). The reflex mechanism of the external sphincter requires integrity of both spinal and cortical pathways. Spinal segments 1–3, the major spinal reflexes necessary for fecal continence, are not affected by Alzheimer's disease, whereas cortical pathways frequently are.

The physiology of continence has been studied experimentally, using balloons to simulate a bolus of feces distending the rectum. In the resting state the internal sphincter (under autonomic involuntary control) maintains a tone sufficient to maintain closure of the anal canal. When a bolus of flatus or feces of sufficient size (150–200 cc) distends the lower rectum, the internal sphincter involuntarily relaxes (the anorectal reflex) (Denny-Brown & Robertson, 1935). The anorectal reflex is similar to receptive relaxation, the mechanism by which a bolus is propelled throughout the entire intestinal tract. When a bolus distends a segment of the intestine, the segment distal to it (further down) relaxes, while the proximal segment contracts to facilitate propulsion through the gut. An intact myenteric plexus is essential for the integrity of the anorectal reflex.

On entering the rectum, the distending mass of flatus or feces stimulates the anorectal reflex. The nerve endings in the richly innervated anoderm, lying within the internal sphincter, are exposed to the distend-

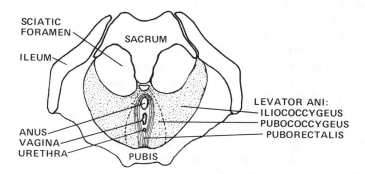

FIGURE 1.2 Relationships of perianal muscular support: caudal view (see text for further details).

ing mass. These nerve endings permit discrimination between solid, liquid, and gas. As a part of the anorectal reflex, the external sphincter contracts at the same time that the internal sphincter relaxes, maintaining continence. This is reinforced by contraction of the pelvic floor muscles to help maintain continence.

If defecation is socially inappropriate following the anorectal reflex, the rectal wall adapts to the presence of the bolus and the rectum now serves as a reservoir for the feces. The internal sphincter returns to its contractile state, inhibiting the desire to defecate (Ihre, 1974). Because the external sphincter can maintain maximal contraction for only 30 to 40 seconds, it relaxes and the internal sphincter continues as the muscle primarily responsible for maintaining continence.

When defecation is socially appropriate, a voluntary increase in intra-abdominal pressure is followed by relaxation of the muscles of the pelvic floor, the anorectal angle is straightened, and defecation occurs.

Causes of Fecal Incontinence

Abnormalities at any level of this system leading to sensory or motor deficits can impair continence and cause incontinence (Figure 1.3). First, neuronal degeneration occurs, with secondary myopathic changes in the sphincters and the levator ani (Parks et al., 1966; Parks et al., 1977; Percy et al., 1982). Degeneration of the myenteric plexus has also been shown in patients with histories of 30 to 40 years of laxative abuse (especially with senna compounds), and in mice experimentally, given prolonged laxative treatment (Smith B, 1968). Excessive use of anticholinergics and phenothiazines can also produce toxic damage to the plexus (Smith B, 1972).

These local neuronal changes (peripheral neuropathy) cause laxity of the sphincter muscles and the levator ani, and the anus becomes patulous. Voluntary contraction of the external sphincter becomes weak. Tone in the puborectalis muscle is decreased and the pelvic floor falls, leading to loss of angulation and impaired efficiency of the flap-valve mechanism (Smith RG, 1983).

In addition to local neuronal damage, abnormalities of the spinal reflex arc mechanism, as in spinal stenosis, tumors, or other space-occupying lesions, can impair the sphincter mechanism. Clinical experience suggests that muscle relaxants such as benzodiazepines can also impair sphincter function.

Second, surgical or obstetrical trauma, or perhaps aging per se, may lead to loss of muscular tone of the levator ani and/or external sphincter. As with neuronal degeneration, this may cause a loss of the anorectal angle and impair external sphincter function.

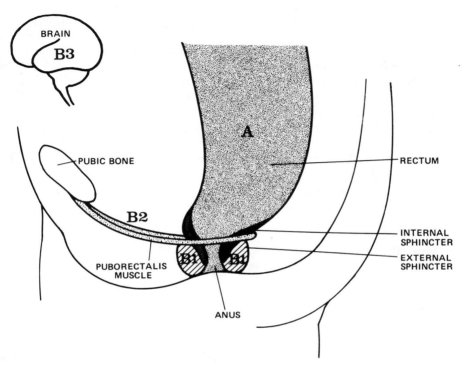

FIGURE 1.3 Fecal soiling. Factors that may result in fecal soiling are: (1) fecal impaction (**A**); (2) impairment of continence mechanisms— impairment of sensory and/or reflex transmission of neuronal stimuli (**B1**), muscular impairment (loss of sphincter tone or anorectal angle) (**B2**), and central nervous system disease (**B3**).

Third, the brain also affects continence. Loss of central voluntary inhibition of the defecation reflex occurs, analogous to the uninhibited neurogenic bladder. Because of cortical deficits, Alzheimer patients may lose voluntary (subconscious) control of the continence mechanism.

Brocklehurst studied 10 patients with fecal incontinence, seven of whom had dementia. In a brief report of this work, the author noted that six patients passed a balloon placed in the rectum before it was fully distended (five of these patients had dementia, the sixth had right hemiplegia). He concluded that elderly patients with organic cerebral disease and fecal incontinence were unable to inhibit intrinsic rectal contractions resulting from distention of a balloon in the rectum. This led to evacuation of the balloon. The author postulated that this mechanism leads to passage of formed stool into the bed or clothing, usually once or twice a day, frequently following the gastrocolic reflex (Brocklehurst, 1972).

Maintenance of continence is multifactorial. Interruption or damage to one part of the complex mechanism may be compensated for so that continence may still be maintained. Mild impairment may lead to incontinence of liquid or gas (flatus), but not solid material. With aging, one impairment may occur but may not lead to fecal soiling until the other compensatory mechanisms are stressed. Thus patients may be able to maintain continence with solid stools, but substantial leakage of liquid feces may occur. Any condition that causes diarrhea (Table 1.7) may overcome the patient's reserve capacity to maintain continence, thereby causing fecal incontinence.

Medical Evaluation

Medical evaluation is needed to identify conditions leading to fecal soiling, including those causing constipation, diarrhea, and impairment of continence.

History A careful medical history (Table 1.8) will usually identify the etiology(ies) for incontinence and suggest strategies for management. A thorough evaluation for conditions causing constipation or diarrhea is essential (see Tables 1.6 and 1.7). The caregiver record (Figure 1.4) provides additional data. Based on the initial history, the record is adapted to the needs of the individual caregiver. After a two-week baseline period, the record is reviewed. Frequently information about fecal pattern, medication, and diet is obtained that was not gathered previously, even with careful questioning. In many situations, use of the caregiver record has enabled the caregiver to identify a pattern and develop an effective management strategy for the problems. Clinical

---

TABLE 1.7 Causes of Diarrhea

I. Motility Disorders
    A. Diverticular disease
    B. Medications
    C. Irritable bowel syndrome
II. Ischemic Colitis
III. Inflammatory Disorders
    A. Acute infections
    B. Inflammatory bowel disease
    C. Diverticulitis

TABLE 1.8 History, Focusing on Fecal Soilage

I. Symptoms
  A. Chronicity (duration)
  B. Stooling pattern (frequency, consistency)
  C. Pain
  D. Bleeding
  E. Continence questions
    1. awareness of passing gas or stool
    2. discrimination between gas, liquid, and solid
    3. leakage (amount, frequency)
    4. accidents (timing)
    5. deferral time (ability to reach commode or bathroom on time)
II. Medical Diseases
  A. Medical conditions producing neuropathy or impairment of muscular function
  B. Past medical history
    1. surgery
    2. trauma
    3. childbirth
III. Medications (Prescription and Over-the-Counter)
  A. Constipation-inducing
    1. anticholinergics
    2. narcotics
    3. iron
    4. diuretics
    5. aluminum-containing antacids
  B. Diarrhea-inducing
    1. cathartics (milk of magnesia, magnesium citrate, Ex-lax)
    2. enemas
    3. magnesium-containing antacids
IV. Diet
  A. Fiber
  B. Fruits
  C. Vegetables
  D. Fluids
V. Environment
  A. Access
    1. restraints or bedrails that inhibit mobility
    2. location of bathroom or commode not remembered by patient
  B. Clothing (patient unable to unfasten clothing adequately)
  C. Caregiver burden (impact of soiling on caregiver)
VI. Caregiver Record (see Figure 1.4)

experience suggests that when caregivers complete such a record, they often feel able to manage the situation.

Physical Examination A routine physical examination is performed, emphasizing evidence of local neuropathy (i.e., anal wink and sphincter tone) (Table 1.9). A routine rectal examination identifies rectal

	Date	Date	Date	Date	Date	Date	Date	Date
Diet								
Fluids								
Fiber								
Stool								
Soilage Y or N								
Amount Small (S) Medium (M) Large (L)								
Consistency Hard (H) Soft (S) Liquid (L)								
Time								
Bowel Medications Enema (E) Suppository (S) Pills (P) Liquid (L)								
Amount or dosage								
Time								
Exercise								
Comments								

FIGURE 1.4 Caregiver record.

contents. Voluntary contraction of the external sphincter is elicited; this may be difficult, however, in cognitively impaired, poorly cooperative patients. In such cases, performing the rectal examination with the patient in the lithotomy position may be helpful. After inserting the examining finger and before palpating the prostate (if the patient is male), the examiner asks the patient to squeeze against the examining finger. If no voluntary contraction follows, the bulbocavernous reflex

TABLE 1.9 Physical Examination, Focusing on Fecal Soilage

I. Abdominal Examination
II. Anorectal Examination
   A. Inspection for mucosal prolapse or procidentia
   B. Sphincter tone
   C. Rule out mass, impaction
   D. Occult blood
III. Neuromuscular Examination
   A. Voluntary external sphincter contraction
   B. Anal reflexes (anal wink and bulbocavernous)
IV. Endoscopic Examination
   A. Indications for endoscopic evaluation need to be considered in the context of the demented patient.
   B. Anoscopy with sensory evaluation can identify whether sensitivity to light touch and pain are intact. In addition, anoscopy is useful to identify fissures, fistulae, tumors, hemorrhoids, and other pathology in the anal canal.
   C. Sigmoidoscopy is used to examine the rectum and rectosigmoid to rule out tumors, inflammation, or diverticular disease.
   D. Colonoscopy is used to rule out tumors, inflammation, diverticular disease, and ischemic bowel disease.

(which can also substitute for the anal wink) may be elicited in the male by applying pressure to the glans penis and waiting for a reflex contraction of the anal sphincter and bulbocavernous muscle. In the female, the appropriate technique is to put a mild traction on the labia majora, thereby compressing the clitoris. The presence of a bulbocavernous reflex signifies an intact reflex arc in the region of the sacral cord. Neuromuscular examination may reveal loss of reflexes.

Laboratory Evaluation Studies should be tailored to confirm the diagnosis suggested by the history and physical examination. As with any medical condition, the laboratory evaluation is individualized for the patient. When causes of diarrhea are suspected, a complete blood count, gram stain, and culture of the stool and a serum titer for *Clostridium difficile* may be indicated. An abdominal radiograph may reveal feces and colonic or rectal distention. Barium enema or endoscopy may be indicated if mechanical obstruction or inflammatory disease are suggested by the history. When transit time must be documented, a barium-containing capsule can be traced radiologically through the gastrointestinal tract. In nondemented patients fecal soilage is an indication for a complete evaluation, including endoscopy and diagnostic imaging. In the demented patient, issues of risk vs. benefit analysis and quality of life need to be taken into consideration when determining the extent of the workup and/or treatment.

Treatment

Despite the frequent presence of a multifactorial etiology for fecal incontinence in Alzheimer patients, clinical experience suggests that treatment for constipation and fecal impaction is the first line of therapy for these patients. The goal of treatment is to have fecal evacuation occur at predictable times, to minimize fecal soiling, and to reduce caregiver burden (see also Burnside, Chapter 2). Treatment of fecal soilage secondary to impaction has two overlapping phases: initial therapy and maintenance therapy. The initial treatment (Table 1.10) focuses on the elimination of precipitating causes, such as constipating or laxative medications. For patients who cannot get to the bathroom on time because of fecal urgency or mobility problems, a commode is recommended. Frequently Alzheimer patients have difficulty with buttons and zippers. Jogging pants with elastic waistbands or velcro closures can facilitate undressing and may eliminate fecal soilage. Attention to the need for privacy is also important for this very personal bodily function.

If these measures are not adequate to resolve the problem, the colon should be emptied of feces. For hard stool, it is best to begin with oil-retention enemas (100–200 cc), followed by daily phosphate enemas or bisacodyl suppositories for up to two weeks. For soft stool, daily phosphate enemas are administered initially. As the lower rectum is emptied, more feces descend and these, too, must be removed or fecal soilage will recur. A two-week course of enemas or suppositories may be necessary to sufficiently clean out the bowel.

It is recommended that, when possible, enema treatment be done by professional personnel. Fluid and electrolyte balance may need to be monitored, especially during the first few days of treatment. Furthermore, the regimen is difficult to manage at home because of increased fecal soilage, especially at the beginning of treatment. Caregivers of incontinent patients are often already stretched to their limits. If patients

---

TABLE 1.10 Fecal Soilage—Initial Therapy

   I. Eliminate Predisposing Factors
      A. Constipating agents
      B. Cathartics
  II. Improve Environment
      A. Commode
      B. Clothing
 III. Remove Stool Accumulation
      A. Hard stool
         1. oil retention enema (100–200 cc olive oil)
         2. daily phosphate enemas (7–14 days)
      B. Soft stool
         1. daily phosphate enemas (7–14 days)

---

are in a respite program or admitted to the acute hospital for other reasons, fecal impaction can easily be treated in these settings. After the first few days or when fecal soilage is minimal, treatment can be completed at home. For patients who must remain at home, visiting nurses can be used for one to two weeks to complete these treatments.

At the same time initial therapy is begun a maintenance program to minimize recurrence can be instituted (Table 1.11). Once the clinician is certain that no obstruction is present, bulk is added to the diet. Dietary fiber increases stool bulk and size because of its water-holding capacity. It decreases transit time, increases gastrointestinal motility, and stimulates peristalsis (American Dietetic Association, 1981). A beginning daily dose of one tablespoon of bran or its equivalent is suggested. If no abdominal cramping or flatulence (excess gas) occurs, the dose can be increased by 1 tablespoon every three to five days until a reasonable stooling pattern is established. WASA HiFiber crackers contain 26% dietary fiber and are available in supermarkets. For most patients, one to three crackers per day will produce one soft stool daily. For patients who are particular about what they eat, WASA crackers are usually acceptable with cheese, butter, or jelly. A liquid beverage can be offered at the same time. Patients can be encouraged to dunk the crackers to moisten them, because the crackers may be too dry and scratchy alone in the mouth. To minimize constipation, fluid intake of 2 liters per day is desirable unless contraindicated by other medical conditions. Only when fluid intake is adequate should bulking agents such as psyllium hydrophilic muciloid be considered. Each teaspoon of psyllium should be taken with at least 8 oz of water to prevent impaction. For patients with persistently hard feces, stool softeners can be added (dioctyl sodium succinate [DSS] up to 500 mg per day). Patients can also be encouraged to increase their intake of fruits and vegetables and to walk as much as possible.

TABLE 1.11 Fecal Soilage Maintenance Therapy

I. Increase Transit Time
  A. Bulk
  B. Bran 20–40 gm, 1 tbsp, increase at 3–5 days as needed
  C. WASA crackers
  D. Psyllium muciloid (1 tsp in 8 oz water twice a day)
  E. Exercise
  F. Consider cathartic or osmotic agents (senna prunes or senna compounds 1–2 tabs at bedtime, lactulose 15–30 cc twice a day)
II. Avoid Constipation
  A. Fluids (2 liters)
  B. Planned evacuation
  C. Daily suppositories
  D. Phosphate enemas timed for gastrocolic reflex
III. Caregiver Record

If mild colonic stimulation is needed, senna (one or two tablets at bedtime or prunes stewed in senna tea), or lactulose (15–30 cc, twice a day) can be used (Brocklehurst et al., 1983). Cathartics such as milk of magnesia, magnesium citrate, cascara, and phenolphthalein are to be avoided if possible because their purgative action may be too strong.

When a substantial neurogenic component coexists, local stimulation of the anal sphincter may be needed to provoke evacuation. To the maintenance regimen described above, a glycerin or bisacodyl suppository can be given at a consistent time daily or every other day to facilitate a planned evacuation. An effective regimen to take advantage of the gastrocolic reflex is to give the suppository just after the patient awakes, or about one-half hour before breakfast. The patient then sits on the commode or goes to the toilet after breakfast.

The effect of treatment can be monitored using the caregiver record (Figure 1.4). Although, theoretically, patients with Alzheimer's disease would be expected to have neurogenic incontinence as a result of their cortical deficits, fecal elimination often becomes predictable and manageable by treating constipation and/or impaction and providing local stimulation with suppositories. For those few patients with neurogenic incontinence for whom this regimen is unsuccessful, the literature suggests alternating constipating agents, such as diphenoxylate hydrochloride or opiates, with enemas or senna derivatives to establish a manageable pattern (Jarrett & Exton-Smith, 1960).

Treatments such as biofeedback (which use operant conditioning to improve sensory awareness of the stimulus) (Wald, 1981), rectal distention (Cerulli et al., 1979), and Kegel exercises to strengthen the pubococcygeus muscle (Kegel, 1956) have been effective in nondemented patients but do not appear to have been studied in Alzheimer patients. Surgery to repair anatomic abnormalities represents a last resort. In most cases the risk/benefit ratio of this form of surgery makes it inappropriate for demented patients.

SUPPORT FOR CAREGIVERS

In treating patients with Alzheimer's disease, physicians must also treat the caregivers (see also Brody, Chapter 6; Tune et al., Chapter 7). The skills and capabilities of the primary caregiver should be assessed at the initial evaluation and reassessed at regular intervals throughout the course of the disease. Physical and emotional health, coping skills, and social and financial resources should be objectively assessed to ensure that the primary caregiver is competent, willing, and able to provide adequate care. Other caregiving arrangements are needed if severe deficiencies in any of these areas are identified. As the disease progresses more care is required from the caregiver. His or her health and expertise should be commensurate with the demand (Council on Scientific Affairs, 1986). The overall medical management plan must include education of caregivers about management of conditions such as insomnia, immobility, and incontinence; knowledge of environmental- and behavioral-management techniques; and information about available resources. Ongoing assessment of specific problem behaviors provides the basis for offering supportive counseling to stressed caregivers. For example, confused patients sometimes wander off for extended periods of time, placing themselves in hazard and greatly alarming their caregivers. A wide variety of devices have been developed in response to this problem, including magnetized plastic strips, attached to clothing, that trigger an alarm beyond a specified exit and digital coded locks. Counseling about use of such devices can help a caregiver allow the patient independent activity within certain "safe" environments without undue fear. The Los Angeles Chapter of ADRDA has instituted a special registry and bracelet program to help caregivers locate a lost person. Undoubtedly, other community groups will develop similar programs.

The support system for the patient and caregivers should be assessed early in the course of the disease and reassessed throughout its progression (see also Tune et al., Chapter 7). Support systems have variable components, including the nature of the relationships and the capability and availability of individuals involved. The patient has substantial care needs; in addition, the primary caregiver may need psychological support, respite, and financial aid. The complexity of the needed support and variability of what each person can provide has to be determined. The data about the support system is usually gathered, over time, by the members of the health professional team from the patient, family, and friends. An example of a compilation of these data is shown in Table 1.12. These data are usually gathered clinically as part of a social history. When assessing the nature of the relationships, the type of emotional and psychological bond between the Alzheimer patient and the primary caregiver is important. Availability includes components such as where the individual lives, his or her reliability, and the nature of the support the individual can provide, for example, transportation or phone calls. Capability includes the individual's own health, finances, and other commitments such as jobs and other family needs.

The relationships depicted are complex and may affect differentially the patient and/or the primary caregiver. For example, the daughter living 500 miles away and working full-time as a bank vice-president has a strong positive relationship with her mother. She provides emotional support through several phone calls each week and ongoing financial

TABLE 1.12 Social Support Network for Alzheimer Patient

Relationship	Age	Living with patient	Nature of bond to: patient	Nature of bond to: caregiver	Distance	Frequency and type of contacts	Health, finances, and other commitments
Mother	96	No	Medium	Weak	5 mi.	Monthly calls	Nursing home resident; no money
Brother	72	No	Medium	Medium	75	Occasional calls	Very sick; some financial help
Sister	70	No	Very strong	Strong	20	Monthly visits; brings food; weekly calls	Not healthy; only small gifts
Daughter	50	No	Very strong	Medium	500	Daily calls; one weekend monthly total care	Strong financial support; important job; busy
Son	48	Sometimes	Medium		0	Responsible for health aide; 3 weekends monthly total care	Manages patient's daily care
Daughter-in-law	52	Sometimes	Weak	Very strong	0	Some cooking, cleaning, transportation, etc.	Helping husband; not employed
Grandson	23	No	Medium	Strong	2,000	Occasional calls to caregiver (father)	Graduate student
Grandson	25	No	Strong	Weak	500	Occasional calls to patient	Full-time job; young children
Granddaughter-in-law	21	No	Weak	Weak	500	No contact	Cares for young children
Friend	73	No	Strong	Strong	3	Daily visits; some cooking; transportation	Healthy, own family far away
Neighbor	68	No	Strong	Strong	0	Some cooking; biweekly visits	Not extremely healthy
Home Health Aide	43	Yes	Medium	Medium	0	Paid employee; 5 days/week; personal care and household chores	Responsible and fairly competent
Clergyman	52	No	Medium	Medium	15	Bimonthly visits	Large congregation; not top priority

support. The son, who lives three miles away, is the primary caregiver. He is somewhat estranged from his mother, but provides all the tangible ongoing support because of his geographic proximity. The son's wife has a minimal emotional bond with the patient but helps because of her relationship with her husband, the primary caregiver. The son gets psychological support from both his wife and his sister.

A family tree (Figure 1.5), based on the type of clinical data detailed in Table 1.12, can help health professionals visualize and make concrete the support network among the Alzheimer patient, the primary caregiver, family, and friends. As additional information is gathered, the figure can be modified. The table lists the type of information usually gathered clinically, but does not have to be completed to use the tree structure. Indeed the figure is best completed over time as additional information is gathered. The family tree, which considers these three components—the nature of the relationship, availability, and capability—can be used as a helpful clinical tool but not as a scientific measure.

The physical and emotional demands of caring for Alzheimer patients can lead to both medical and psychiatric illnesses in the caregivers. Depression has been documented, with recent data suggesting that depressive disorders are found in a striking one-third to one-half of caregivers of homebound frail elders (Gallagher et al., in press; Rabins et al., 1982; Barnes et al., 1981). Caregivers may ignore their own medical needs, allowing mild illnesses like congestive heart failure and hypertension to progress to symptomatic states. Clinical experience indicates that caregivers can develop acute medical illnesses, which sometimes require hospitalization. This hospitalization often leads to a crisis in caregiving for the Alzheimer patient.

Another aspect of medical problems of caregivers is drug use. Careful questioning of caregivers about medications may uncover inappropriate drug use to cope with their own medical and psychiatric conditions, which are in need of treatment. When patients with Alzheimer's disease are treated with drugs such as sedative hypnotics, caregivers sometimes use the patient's medications to relieve their own symptoms of anxiety and insomnia. A supportive rather than punitive approach with such a caregiver can guide him or her into substance abuse treatment programs. Alleviating caregiver burden by appropriate referrals to social support services can help remove the underlying impetus to drug use.

SUMMARY

Preserving remaining abilities, identifying treatable conditions, supporting caregivers, and managing specific syndromes are the mainstays of medical management of Alzheimer patients. Primary-care physicians and

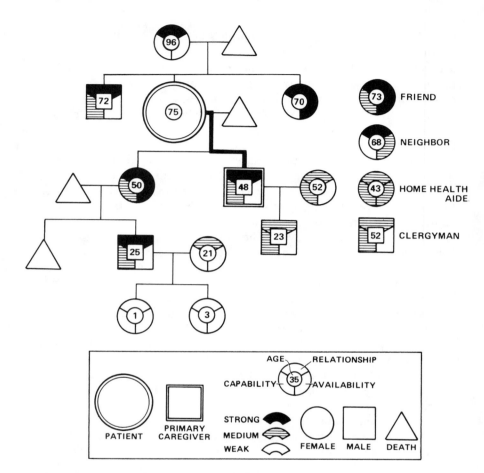

FIGURE 1.5 Social support network for Alzheimer patient.

specialists can improve the quality of life for these patients and their caregivers by developing appropriate management strategies.

The author wishes to acknowledge the following grant support: NIMH Research Grant MN-40041, Subproject #4, NIH-NIA Research Grant 5K08 A G00246, and the Veterans Administration. The opinions expressed herein are those of the author and not necessarily those of the Veterans Administration.

The author wishes to thank T. Franklin Williams, M.D., Eric Larson, M.D., Mary Goldstein, M.D., Susan Cottle, M.S.W., Meghan Gerety, M.D., Donald Peck, M.D., and Donald Bliwise, M.D. for their perceptive comments and critiques that added enormously to the quality of this chapter. I also wish to thank Butch Colyear for his patience and artistic talent in preparing the artwork.

2
Nursing Care

Irene Burnside

"It is time for us to trust our experience and judgment, time to experiment systematically with new methods. Many of our old ways to deal with dementia were based on ignorance."

(Rader, Doan, & Schwab, 1985)

Nurses have long provided care for demented persons, and their experiences have often been poignant ones (Breeze, 1909). Nurses' involvement during the long downhill trajectory of Alzheimer's disease covers a wide range of services, reflecting the need for complex and holistic care.

This chapter will cover a variety of issues involved in providing nursing care for the Alzheimer patient. The underlying perspective is fourfold: (1) the individual with Alzheimer's must be viewed as a biological, psychological, and social being, requiring holistic treatment; (2) the care plan must be modified as the individual progresses through worsening phases of the disease (Reisberg, 1984), with self-care encouraged until impairment prevents it (Eliopoulos, 1984; Hirschfeld, 1985; Lantz, 1985; Orem, 1985); (3) nursing practice must be guided by the fundamental principle of maximizing stability for patients (Hall, 1983); and (4) care must be given in the most humane way possible.

PHASES OF NURSING CARE IN ALZHEIMER'S DISEASE

Each phase of Alzheimer's disease presents unique problems for the nursing profession. As the patient's disability increases, appropriate assessments must be made to insure his or her safety and well-being as well as that of others. Ongoing evaluation of both patient and environment is essential and provides the basis for numerous decisions about the kind and level of care required. Various authors have written about nursing management of Alzheimer patients (Jones IH, 1979; Pinel, 1975; Powter, 1977; Burnside, 1979; Hayter, 1974).

Even during the relatively early stage of Alzheimer's disease, when dementia is moderate, evaluation must be made of the patient's level of disorientation, since it determines to a large extent the person's ability to carry out activities of daily living. Self-care abilities should also be assessed so that the amount of assistance needed can be gauged. Cognitive impairment does not necessarily correlate exactly with impairment of self-care. For example, some patients, despite severe disorientation, are able to dress themselves (Winograd, 1984). As much independence as possible should be encouraged. Since bathing and personal hygiene often present problems at this stage of Alzheimer's disease, careful assessment is essential in these areas.

As dementia becomes moderately severe, the nursing plan must reflect decreases in the patient's abilities to provide self-care. Dressing may now require assistance. Fear of bathing may develop. Urinary and later fecal incontinence may ensue. There may be displays of "sundowning" (see discussion later in this chapter). The patient may develop a tendency to wander. This functional decline and decreased ability to perform tasks of daily living and to interact socially can present major nursing problems. Seizures, too, may begin to occur and may cause alarm in caregivers, especially if they have not been warned that they could occur. Ongoing, periodic reevaluation is essential to revise nursing plans according to the patient's changing needs (see also Winograd, Chapter 1).

The late, or severe, phase of Alzheimer's disease demands exquisite nursing care to prevent infections, bedsores, and contractures. By this phase the patient has limited speech and has lost motor abilities. The importance of nonverbal communication becomes paramount. The late-phase patient is likely, however, to be unresponsive to attempts at communication, frustrating caregivers. Greater emphasis must, therefore, be placed on keeping up caregiver strength and morale.

It should be noted that nursing care is difficult when a patient is totally incompetent and unresponsive. The terminal phase may be very short, or it may be prolonged, in part by nursing care. Preventions of infections, injury to self, starvation, and fluid and electrolyte imbalance are some of the major concerns of nurses during this phase. As Wolanin and Phillips (1981) say, "Although it is tempting to forget the patient is a person, the assumption must be made that the unresponsive body and mind are receiving the messages sent to them by gentle touch, warm hands, kind voices, refreshing cold drinks, soothing warm baths and massage, dry clean beds and the comfort of position changes" (p. 345).

It is important to prevent burnout in all caregivers, whether family members or nursing staff. This is not the time to decrease the amount of support for the family members. Special care and attention should be taken to monitor the attitudes and caring abilities of ancillary and nursing personnel. This chapter focuses on nursing care, primarily for institutionalized patients. Aspects of this care can be incorporated into community- or hospital-based nursing care and can be appropriately taught to nonprofessional caregivers (see also Tune et al., Chapter 7).

ASSESSMENT OF ALZHEIMER PATIENTS

Physical Assessment

In the physical assessment, the nurse checks vital signs, lungs, heart, bowel sounds, skin, and extremities. The nurse will gather data on which to base nursing diagnoses and an individualized nursing care plan. There may be alterations in exercise and activity related to the patient's muscle strength and joint motion. Or there may be an altered bowel and bladder pattern, leading to impaction and dehydration: the goal is to maintain bowel and bladder continence for as long as possible. Baseline data are crucial. The nurse will also gather data about altered nutritional patterns. Patients sometimes forget to eat or to drink fluids. Because aging skin is often dry, dehydration may not be considered a serious problem. It is important that this portion of the physical examination not be over-looked. A nursing care plan for adequate hydration and diet is needed. Altered sleep and rest patterns are other components of the nursing database. Wandering behavior and sundowning will need special nursing orders. In both the physical and mental assessments the nurse must confirm the data with family or other caregivers. Because of cognitive changes, the patient is not always a reliable informant.

Mental Assessment

Because there will be altered cognitive and perceptual abilities, the nurse must also make a mental assessment. Confusion and disorientation of Alzheimer patients needs to be dealt with by the nursing staff (Nowa-kowski, 1985; Patrick, 1967; Wolanin, 1984). The mental status of the patient can be assessed by screening instruments such as Pfeiffer's Portable Mental Status Questionnaire (Pfeiffer, 1975); Folstein's Mini-

Mental State Examination (Folstein et al., 1975) (see Appendix 1); and the Mental Status Questionnaire (Kahn et al., 1960).

Cognitive decline can also be assessed by asking patients to draw a clock or write their name. (See Figure 2.1.) Behrendt (1984) states that, "Just before complete loss of writing ability, an Alzheimer patient will reach a condition where he or she will be unable to write or sign their name on command. If the name is placed before them, however, the patient will proceed to write. It appears that in some instances the patient is unable to write without a model because they are unable to remember the order in which the letters occur. Other patients, however, are unable to remember the construction of the various letters appearing in their name" (p. 88).

When assessing mental status the nurse needs to be aware of the fact

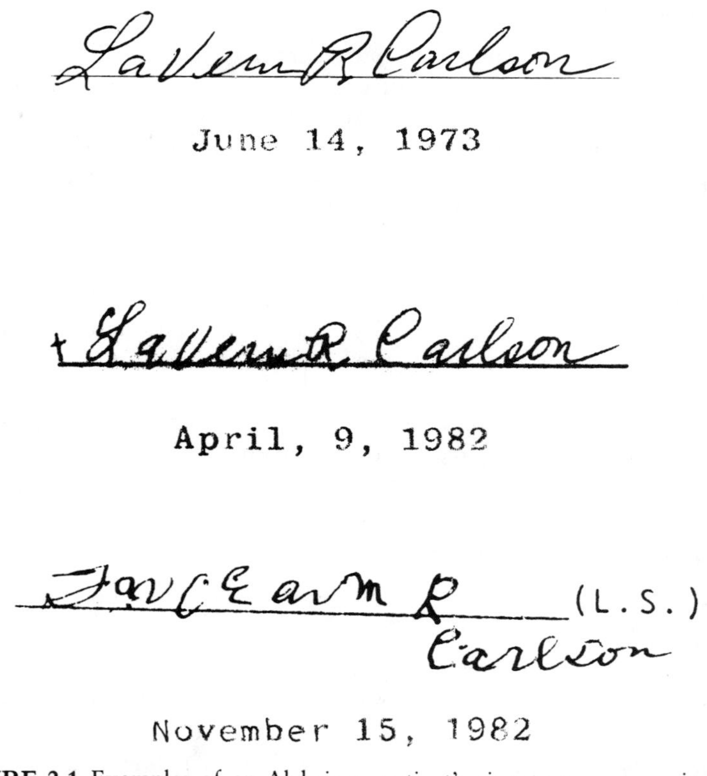

June 14, 1973

April, 9, 1982

(L.S.)

November 15, 1982

FIGURE 2.1 Examples of an Alzheimer patient's signatures over a nine-year period. Notice the rapid deterioration of the ability to write a signature from April to November.

that some patients may socialize well despite major cognitive impairment. Other patients may function poorly in the social realm with relatively intact cognition. Depression can also mimic dementia and is common in conjunction with Alzheimer's disease (see also, Winograd, Chapter 1; Satlin & Cole, Chapter 3; Cohen, Chapter 5; Tune et al., Chapter 7).

Psychosocial assessment has great relevance for planning care and should be given as much importance as physical assessment. Previous hobbies and interests, as well as relationships to (or interest in) pets (Erickson, 1985), can provide guidelines for optimal care. Participating in familiar activities is often helpful for an Alzheimer patient. Memory aids and maintaining consistent routines may enable the patient to function better (Table 2.1) (see also Winograd, Chapter 1).

TABLE 2.1 Memory Aids

(Note: Many of these aids are appropriate for patients with or without help in the earlier phases of Alzheimer's disease. Later they may have to be done for the patient. Others are appropriately used by caregivers at all phases of the disease. Patients should be encouraged and helped to do as much self-care as possible.)

I. General
   A. Keep pen and white, undecorated paper for reminder notes in same place for easy location. (Use black felt tipped pen if visual impairment exists)
   B. Simplify activity schedule.
   C. Place easily read list of important numbers near telephone, most used ones first.
   D. Keep doctor's instructions for taking medication and other health care in visible, consistent place (e.g., post on wall or refrigerator door).
   E. Keep checklist near the usual exit door of things to be done before leaving house (e.g., put keys in pocket, turn off stove, put out the cat, lock door).

II. Daily Activities
   A. Make a checklist of daily activities with times in large print. Keep in visible and consistent place.
   B. Set alarm clock or a timer as reminder of specific things to be done. Place note by clock or timer reminding of what is to be done.
   C. Arrange to have a friend call at designated times to remind of an appointment.
   D. Establish consistent routines for important activities (e.g., put morning medication near pan used to cook morning cereal).

III. Location
   A. Remind person of where he or she is, or is going, and why.
   B. Place signs designating important locations such as bathroom.
   C. Place pictures designating function on refrigerator, stove, bathroom door.

(continued)

TABLE 2.1 Memory Aids (*continued*)

D. Keep person's familiar, significant objects in consistent locations.
E. Post list of major items in each cupboard and drawer.
F. Arrange for a friend to become familiar with objects in the home to help if they are misplaced.
G. Attach eye glasses to a chain that the person can wear around the neck.
IV. Wandering
    A. Use identification necklace or necklace with name and address that patient cannot remove.
    B. Attach name and address of patient on strips of cloth that can be put on back of clothing with velcro.
    C. Alert police and neighbors to the person's possible need for assistance in finding the way home.
    D. Keep card in the person's wallet or purse or taped to jacket or hat with directions to home and name and telephone number of responsible person.
    E. Enroll patient in a special registry program where available, e.g., the Los Angeles Chapter of ADRDA has instituted a special registry and bracelet program that allows for the registry of persons suffering from chronic memory loss. The patient will wear a bracelet with a code number, his first name, the words "Memory Loss," and a central telephone number. The code will be registered on a computer maintained by ADRDA.
    F. Use structured activity programs to help reduce wandering.
    G. Use buddy system in institutional settings to help patients watch one another.
    H. Use fenced-in yards and buzzer systems to alert staff or caregivers that a patient is wandering.
    I. Establish a protocol for all staff members to use when patient wanders off.
    J. Conduct frequent in-service classes about management of wanderers.

Environmental Assessment

Nurses need to assess carefully the environment of Alzheimer patients, both in acute hospital and chronic care facilities (Palmer, 1983). The optimal environment provides a safe, secure and stable milieu, while at the same time promoting freedom and stimulation. Nurses have become very aware of environmental factors in dealing with Alzheimer patients (Cox, 1985; Schafer, 1985; Peppards, 1985; Whall & Conklin, 1985).

A wide variety of details must be attended to in assessing patient safety. Stability requires that routines, personnel, and furniture remain as consistent as possible. The pragmatics of the day-to-day care of Alzheimer patients in many different environments have been written about

(Burnside, 1982a, 1982b; Burnside & Moehrlin, 1980; Mackey, 1983). Nurses must assess the patient's environment for problem areas that may be adding to his or her disorientation and distress. Necessary emotional stimulation must be provided. It is important to create an atmosphere of freedom and mobility and avoid use of restraints (DiFabio, 1981; Yarmesch & Sheafor, 1984). Thorough assessment of the care environment and the implementation of good environmental designs are a major element in providing adequate and humane nursing care for Alzheimer sufferers (see Table 2.2).

Communication

Assessment of patients' communication skills can guide programs and procedures to enhance the quality of life for Alzheimer victims. It is important that nonverbal communication be included in both evaluation and treatment plans. The ability to communicate varies from patient to patient and usually decreases gradually as Alzheimer's disease progresses. Even when individuals cannot communicate very well, if they are outgoing and pleasant they may function well in a daycare setting. They can either observe or be a group member, even though they cannot carry on sustained conversations or interact for long with one person. The basics of communication (Bartol, 1979; Burnside, 1980a, 1981) underscore the need to understand and value nonverbal communication with Alzheimer patients, especially during the more advanced phases. Communication, both nonverbal and verbal, is also important in the group context (Baker, 1985; Schwab et al., 1985; Burnside et al., 1984; Burnside, 1984, 1985).

Little has been written about the friendship between people with severe cognitive impairments, or about how they communicate with one another. Over the years this writer has observed numerous friendships between impaired people who do not talk rationally with one another but carry on conversations as they walk together. They seem to select someone with approximately the same level of impairment and appear to find warmth and comfort in their close alliance. When the friendship occurs between a man and a woman, staff members may discourage it. Spouses are sometimes jealous and may even transfer the loved one to another facility. Some spouses, however, are able to understand and support the meaning of these relationships (Burnside, 1981).

Many caregivers find it difficult to interact with patients whose verbal skills are impaired. It is even more difficult to interpret and respond to nonverbal cues. Along with assessment of the patient's limitation in communication, nurses need to develop confidence in their own

TABLE 2.2 Environmental Aids

  I. Safety
   A. Use combination locks on doors between wards or to the outside.
   B. Dismantle bathroom door locks to prevent patients from locking themselves in.
   C. Make sure floors are not highly polished to prevent falls.
   D. Wipe up spills and urine immediately.
   E. Avoid candles and artificial fruit that can be mistaken for food.
   F. Adjust water temperature in faucets to avoid scalding.
   G. Keep medications locked up at all times.
   H. Have beds low to the floor.
   I. Have padded tongue blades visible in patients' rooms and recreation areas for use in seizures.
   J. Place signs at patient's bedside or doorway to room, indicating special care needs.
   K. Provide adequate light without glare. Older patients usually require extra light.
   L. Teach all staff members and caregivers the Heimlich method to use if patient chokes.
   M. Place bright tape on bottom step because of depth perception problems.
 II. Stability
   A. Maintain consistent furniture arrangement. Make changes gradually.
   B. Avoid moving patient from one bed or room to another.
   C. Have items familiar to individual in environment and encourage their use.
   D. Maintain predictable daily routines.
   E. Take history of patient's habits. Use as guide for daily activities.
   F. Develop long-term, consistent staff.
   G. Have staff members establish one-to-one relationships with patients.
   H. Avoid entering room suddenly, especially if room is darkened.
   I. Change dressings, dress and undress patients in own room or private area.
   J. Remove or cover large mirrors if patients become agitated by them.
III. Stimulation
   A. Create a cheerful environment using vibrant colors.
   B. Avoid use of light blues and greens with aged patients, as they often have difficulty seeing these colors.
   C. Decorate with visually stimulating objects such as posters, mobiles, pictures, and tropical fish.
   D. Provide large calendars and draw an X through each day to orient patients in time. Large clocks and seasonal decorations also orient patients.
   E. Provide bulletin boards and classes in reality orientation.
   F. Use touch and eye contact as well as words to contact patients.
   G. Encourage visits by family, friends, children, and pets.
   H. Monitor radios, stereos, and TVs for noise levels.
   I. Remove patients from areas of excessive noise and activity.
   J. Introduce reminiscence group therapy in early phases of disease.

(*continued*)

TABLE 2.2 Environmental Aids (*continued*)

IV. Freedom and Mobility
    A. Provide open space so that patients are free to move around.
    B. Avoid light-colored tile floors with dark geometric designs; these confuse patients with faulty perception.
    C. Hand mitts inhibit door opening, tampering with tubes and dressings, and taking other people's property. Can be used instead of restraints.
    D. Place photo and name of patient on door to bedroom.
    E. Paint bathroom and toilet doors in bright colors so that patients can identify them.
    F. Encourage walks as a daily activity.

Source: Adapted from Moehrlin, 1985; Ramsey, 1985; Wolanin & Phillips, 1981; and author.

ability to make comprehensible and useful interventions with verbally impaired patients. Skillful communication with such patients includes being able to use simple sentences and nonverbal cues such as touch, eye contact, and hand gestures. It means being able to sense the patient's feelings and respond to them without offering false reassurance.

Communication between nurse and patient should involve daily one-to-one contact during which the nurse checks the comfort of the patient, explains procedures if necessary, and, whenever possible, aids the patient in establishing contact with others. Out of such contact the nurse can gain a more precise understanding of the patient's needs, that is, level of supervision, adjustments in amount and nature of stimulation, and shifts in routines. Table 2.3 suggests appropriate nursing interventions to improve communication with the demented patient. These interventions are based on observation of specific behaviors the patient manifests.

SPECIAL CARE NEEDS OF ALZHEIMER PATIENTS

Elimination

Nursing is the one discipline that must deal with elimination 24 hours a day and provide expertise in its management (see also Winograd, Chapter 1). Family members often can manage the care of an Alzheimer patient at home or with respite care until elimination problems begin. Then professional help is needed, sometimes resulting in the patient's institutionalization. Nursing interventions help establish regular elimination patterns and provide patient comfort. Detailed observation of the patient is essential: noticing behaviors that indicate a need to go to the bathroom (e.g., restlessness or fumbling with fly); identifying symptoms that may indicate constipation (e.g., nausea); checking for irrita-

TABLE 2.3 Communicating with Alzheimer Patient

Patient behavior	Nursing intervention
I. *Interpersonal Difficulties*	
A. Patient fails to understand or follow nurse's instructions	Use simple sentences, nonverbal cues.
B. Patient does not respond to simple sentences and nonverbal cues	Allow several seconds for response. If no response, repeat sentence exactly. If still no response, restructure sentence.
C. Patient ignores nurse	Address patient by most familiar name. Touch, move in closer, make eye contact. Ask yes or no questions.
D. Patient looks bewildered	Check your phrasing, tone of voice. Start over, introducing self, saying what you want patient to do, or will do to him or her.
E. Patient walks away, refuses to interact	If patient seems depressed, walk with patient in silence, watch for response (e.g., looking at you, slowing walk, wringing hands). Touch lightly and watch for acceptance or withdrawal.
	If patient seems agitated: leave, stating intention to return in awhile.
F. Patient backs away	Do not move closer. Slow movement and speech. Use small talk to establish trust. Lower voice. Avoid patronizing. Communicate caring.
G. Patient is isolated and does not mingle	Assign staff person for daily one-to-one contact: sitting, talking, walking, having a cup of coffee or tea. Check patient's comfort regularly: clothes, room, skin, fatigue, toilet needs, hunger, thirst. Introduce patient in appropriate size group (not overpowering).

(continued)

TABLE 2.3 Communicating with Alzheimer Patient (*continued*)

Patient behavior	Nursing intervention
II. *Emotional Distress*	
A. Patient exhibits fear	Verbalize patient's feelings, preferably through questioning (e.g., if patient is trembling: "Joe, you are trembling. Are you afraid?").
B. Patient acknowledges fear or anxiety	Acknowledge patient's feelings. Do not offer false reassurance. If in doubt, listen and hold patient's hand.
C. Patient is out of touch with reality (e.g., wants to visit mother, who is dead)	Try once to explain reality. If not accepted, back off to avoid catastrophic reaction. (See discussion in chapter under "Other Problematic Behaviors.")
D. Patient's voice is rising	This indicates agitation and may require putting patient in quiet room. Staff person with best relationship to patient should take over, calm and soothe patient, avoid argument or irritation. Can lead to catastrophic reaction. Attempt diversion.
III. *Verbal Impairment*	
A. Patient substitutes words with similar sounds	If you are sure of correct word, supply it. If not sure, ask patient to point or describe. Avoid correcting patient.
B. Patient substitutes words with similar meanings, e.g., "running machine" for car	Try to guess what patient means. Ask if you are correct.
C. Patient rambles and strings phrases together	Try to make sense of patient's words. Pay attention to nonverbal cues and unspoken feelings.
IV. *Eating Problems*	
A. Patient exhibits poor appetite	Check for depression or paranoia. Explain what meal is, guide

(*continued*)

TABLE 2.3 Communicating with Alzheimer Patient (*continued*)

Patient behavior	Nursing intervention
	patient to utensils, encourage to eat. Allow plenty of time for meal (40 minutes). Offer several small meals each day. Use salt or piquant sauce to stimulate appetite. Avoid dry, scratchy foods. Offer fluids, including liquid diet supplements, between meals. Avoid hard-to-handle foods such as jello, spaghetti, and peas.
B. Patient coughs and chokes during meal	Reduce patient's stimulation, including conversation while eating. Avoid foods at room temperature and liquids, also tough, stringy meats. Give patient verbal cues to swallow. Be sure staff are trained in Heimlich maneuver.
C. Patient is passive during meal	Encourage patient to feed him- or herself. Do not leave patient alone to eat.
D. Patient is confused when in dining room	Try to keep patient in chair without using restraints. Hold patient's hand. Touch patient. Offer only one food at a time. Create soothing environment with cues that this is a pleasant place to eat. Serve desserts separately, after meal has been eaten.

tion caused by wetness; and monitoring the effectiveness of medications and diet. Nurses use a variety of techniques to aid elimination: dietary adjuncts, medications, and human interventions (Table 2.4).

Nutrition

The nutrition of Alzheimer patients needs close monitoring. In either nursing home or hospital settings the patient may be depressed, withdrawn, apathetic, or unwilling to eat. The paranoid patient may think that the food is being poisoned. The aggressive patient may steal food from other patients' trays.

In later phases of the disease, patients often cannot remember having eaten or taken fluids. Someone else must, therefore, organize the feeding routine and keep track of nutrition. Finger foods can help by permitting

TABLE 2.4 Establishing Elimination Patterns

The goal of treatment is to establish regular, predictable elimination, with little or no soiling, while assuring the patient's privacy, comfort, and dignity (see also Winograd, Chapter 1).

Observation	Intervention
A. Patient exhibits urinary or fecal incontinence	Take history of bladder and bowel function. Offer bedpan or take patient to bathroom at least every two hours. Do not ask patient to hold either urine or bowel movement. Dress patient in easily removable clothing such as jogging suit or slacks with elastic waistband. Make sure patient has privacy for elimination. Keep patient clean and dry. Use cornstarch in fleshy folds to avoid irritation. Avoid using a blaming tone of voice.
B. Incontinence persists	Provide commode and make sure bed is close to floor. Supply briefs (avoid calling them diapers) that hold liquid away from skin. Monitor effect of treatment closely (see Resnick, 1984; Winograd & Jarvik, 1986; Greengold & Ouslander, 1986, for further discussion of urinary incontinence).
C. Incontinence still persists	With fecal incontinence it may be necessary to empty bowels and regulate elimination with use of enemas and dietary aids.
D. Patient exhibits constipation	Take history of bowel function. Nausea sometimes indicates constipation. Monitor bowel movements and if constipated add bran, dried fruit, or prune juice to diet. Reduce dose when stool becomes too soft or patient has abdominal pain or flatulence. Add bran or other fibers to diet.

(continued)

TABLE 2.4 Establishing Elimination Patterns *(continued)*

Observation	Intervention
E. Constipation persists	If no bowel movement in three days, use glycerin suppository before breakfast, take to bathroom after breakfast. Increase fluid intake. When adequate, add bulking agents to diet. Monitor effects of treatment closely.
F. Constipation still persists	Program of enemas may be needed.

patients to eat without utensils, though families and staff often find this hard to tolerate. Plastic containers may need opening because apractic patients cannot maneuver them. Tough or stringy meats are best avoided, since swallowing becomes difficult. Nurses must work closely with the nutritionist and other staff members to adjust and monitor the nutrition of patients throughout the progression of Alzheimer's disease. A careful food history, including the patient's likes and dislikes, will help in designing an effective nutritional program.

Activity and Exercise

Activity and exercise are important for the general health and well-being of Alzheimer patients. Exercise helps prevent constipation and bedsores. Structured activity programs reduce wandering behaviors and agitation. Although most patients will ultimately need total care, efforts should be made to keep the patient active and involved as long as possible in enjoyable activities. However, the patient should not be forced to participate, since this can damage self-esteem and lead to catastrophic reaction (see discussion later in this chapter under "Other Problematic Behavior"). Assessment of prior lifestyle and activity can serve as a guide in planning exercise and activities.

When patients resist exercise and exhibit lethargic behavior, fatigue may be a cause. Napping can raise the patient's energy level and make him or her more amenable to activity, but in some cases it might lead to nighttime wakefulness. With inactive patients, encouragement by staff is crucial in getting them mobilized. Encouraging patients to help staff with chores, such as gardening and dishwashing, and praising their efforts will increase the patient's activity level. Assisting patients with self-care, rather than doing for them in order to save time, provides exercise and enhances self-esteem. Volunteers and students can play an important role, taking patients for walks or wheelchair rides and playing games with them.

Sundowning

Some Alzheimer patients become active at night, interfering with the sleep of others (Evans, 1985; Huey, 1985). This behavior is known as sundowning. If possible the patient's habits should be reoriented toward greater daytime activity and nighttime rest. Reduction of naps and increase of daytime activities may help. Late afternoon activity, a long walk, for example, may lead to more peaceful nights. Bedtime snacks and hot milk can sometimes aid sleep. Scheduling the heaviest dose of tranquilizers for evening is often useful in repatterning sleep. Environmental influences should be attended to as well: soft lights in the bedroom and soft music on the radio; shades to block out excess light and draperies to block out loud noises; a cool, but not cold, temperature in the room; familiar objects, such as pillow, clock, and photographs; and staff clad in soft colors. All these can be soothing to patients with confusion and anxiety brought on by failing perceptual and cognitive powers. Careful explanation of what is going on may also relax confused or anxious patients. A trip to the bathroom just before bedtime and a bathroom nightlight or bedside commode are also helpful in reducing sundowning. To facilitate night toilet needs, the bed should be placed close to the floor with the rails down, but the patient should be assessed to assure that he or she can stand up safely from a low bed (see also Winograd, Chapter 1).

Wandering Behavior

The wanderers among Alzheimer patients wreak havoc in all settings. Wandering requires constant surveillance to prevent patients from getting lost or hurting themselves. Moreover, wanderers sometimes go into the rooms of others and meddle with their possessions. This creates problems in both nursing homes and daycare centers.

There has been little research on wandering behavior, yet nurses must cope with it. As with so many behavioral problems of Alzheimer patients, the key to management is in the nurse's ability to make contact and to communicate with the patient. This means being able to listen and respond to verbal and nonverbal cues and to know when to come forward and when to back off.

Often when wandering occurs, the patient is playing out a personal agenda. Recognizing that agenda (for example, the patient is worried that her family will not be fed, or the patient feels he has to go home) and responding to it, even repeating words the patient has used, sometimes distract the person from leaving. When this fails, the patient must be accompanied and the nurse should continue attempting to maintain contact, repeating phrases and naming the patient's underlying emotions. Talking directly about the present situation (such as reminding the patient of the rest home or hospital) may calm the person, but sometimes it increases distress. When this occurs, reminders should be dropped. Redirection can also be tried, for example, suggesting, "let's walk this way now." If the patient resists, he or she should be allowed to control the direction, with the nurse accompanying to ensure safety (Rader et al., 1985).

Since wandering can be a dangerous problem in any health care facility, special precautions must be taken to ensure the patients' safety (see Tables 2.1 and 2.2). Space is essential for the maintenance of wanderers' physical health. When the response to wandering is to restrain or constrict patients, they suffer loss of bone mass, decreased mobility, reduction in strength, and impaired balance (Rader et al., 1985).

Clinically, wandering behavior is most noticeable after patients have been relocated or after first-time admission to a hospital or nursing home. The wandering patient seems bent on going home. This pattern alone indicates the need for orientation programs and should alert staff to make greater efforts in making the patient feel welcome. Exquisite care is needed, especially during the first few weeks after admission, until the patient settles in (Burnside, 1980b; Robb, 1985).

Other Problematic Behaviors

Several other behaviors, common in Alzheimer's disease, require assessment and special care. These include catastrophic reactions, aggressive and combative behaviors, paranoia, withdrawal, seizures, and inappropriate sexual behaviors.

Catastrophic Reactions

Catastrophic reactions were described by Goldstein (1969) in his work with brain-damaged soldiers. Under stress the impaired individual responds with intense emotion and may explode in rage or begin suddenly to cry or show signs of high anxiety. Examinations that are too fast or too pressured are typical situations in which catastrophic reactions may occur. Bathing is another high-stress situation for many patients. When a reaction occurs during bathing, leaving the patient alone for a few minutes often eases the tension, and the patient may then be willing to bathe. A stable environment reduces the incidence of catastrophic reactions. Edelson and Lyons (1985) offer excellent suggestions about handling some of the challenging nursing care situations that arise with difficult patients.

Aggressive and Combative Behavior

Aggressive behavior strains a family's coping mechanisms to the hilt. Elderly wives may become frightened of husbands they never before feared. Children are aghast at the violence and abuse they see their parent exhibit. The aggressive person can sometimes be cared for at a daycare center, particularly if there is some use of a mild tranquilizer, but may be almost unmanageable at home. Aggressive behaviors may occur during prolonged assessment procedures and during rituals in nursing homes.

In research about violent incidents by nursing home residents with organic brain dysfunction, Jones MK (1985) found that morning hours are a prime time for outbursts. According to Jones, 28% of all incidents of violence occurred between 9:00 A.M. and 10:00 A.M. This is a time of high activity in any nursing home, involving bathing, feeding, medications, treatments, and doctors' rounds. Also, more incidents occurred on the night shift than on the evening shift. Targets of the violent behaviors were predominantly direct-service staff. Nursing assistants were assaulted 71 times; nurses, 25 times; and nursing students, four times. No doctors were assaulted.

Management of combative and aggressive behaviors is one of the most demanding of nursing functions. It requires calmness, firmness, and a sense of authority. In-service classes on prevention and management, and the development of protocols for dealing with combative patients, can ease the problems nurses face in the immediate situation of violent behavior. As with other behavioral problems, the existence of a one-to-one relationship between the patient and a calm and understanding staff member is the key to management.

Aggressiveness can be mitigated if nurses notice frustration and agitation, which are often precursors to violent acting out. Interactions leading to the frustration and agitation can be curtailed, modified, or slowed down. Sometimes the patient can be diverted. Medication should be checked to make sure that incorrect dosage or side effects are not factors.

When behavior reaches the violent stage it can be accepted only when no one (including the patient) can be hurt. Violent behavior cannot be tolerated in groups, since it frightens other group members. In attempting to quiet a combative patient it is essential to maintain a neutral, nonhostile tone and to avoid overwhelming the patient with too many staff members converging at once. It is always better to have the staff person who relates best to the individual take charge of the situation. Taking the patient to a private room and trying to get the patient to communicate the reason for his or her outburst are the most effective means of quieting a violent patient. When the patient cannot verbalize, the staff person should remain with him or her in a quiet room and attempt to make contact through touch, eye contact, and verbalization.

Paranoid Behaviors

Paranoia is often a component in agitated and aggressive behavior. Sensory impairments, such as visual and hearing loss and decrease in sense of taste and smell, can enhance paranoia, since they render the environment less comprehensible and, therefore, more suspect. Recognizing that paranoia stems from fear of a world that can no longer be fully grasped is a first step in understanding how to manage it. Sometimes wandering and pacing behaviors are indications of agitation in suspicious patients; such behaviors should not be discouraged if they seem to decrease frustration and agitation. Objects that can be used as weapons should, however, be placed out of reach. Full-length mirrors can sometimes be a source of agitation. The patient may strike out either in the belief that the person he or she sees is an impostor or out of dismay at his or her appearance. In extreme cases the mirror should be removed. Frequently covering the mirror with a curtain is adequate (Schwab et al., 1985).

Withdrawal

In the beginning stages of Alzheimer's disease, when the individual becomes aware that something is wrong, withdrawal may be noticed by loved ones. The afflicted person may stop frequenting the local bar with friends. The person may appear depressed. Early identification and assessment can aid in development of useful treatment strategies. Emotional involvement with withdrawn patients is crucial, although often frustrating. The withdrawn patient in the early stages of Alzheimer's disease is often acutely aware of others' responses to him or her and may resist self-exposure.

Seizures

Accurate data are lacking on the number of Alzheimer patients who develop seizures in the later phases of the disease. Family members often are not informed that this may occur and are frightened when they witness a seizure. Sometimes caregivers think that the seizure is related to something they have said or done. Nurses, too, are often not knowledgeable about seizures in Alzheimer patients. There is a need for protocols to be developed so that all staff know how to deal with seizures. Information about the patient's history of seizures and other relevant data should be boldly displayed on the chart, discussed in in-service training, and reported at shift changes.

Sexual Behaviors

Issues of sexual behavior and sexual intimacy are usually absent from descriptions of Alzheimer's disease. Staff members are frequently distressed by sexual behaviors or the lack of modesty they see in patients. The forgetful patient may forget to put on all items of clothing or may not zip a fly. Sometimes sexual overtures to staff members occur. Often they are signs that the individual needs more affection, caring, and touching. Paying attention to the circumstances under which sexual behaviors occur is also important. For example, a staff person who sits down on a bed next to a patient of the opposite sex with hips touching should not be surprised if the patient responds with a sexual gesture.

As verbal communication diminishes, the need for human contact is more often expressed physically. Mute patients who cannot respond to conversations have been known simply to reach over and touch a nurse or kiss her gently on the cheek. When behavior is more overtly sexual or when nudity is involved, staff members who remain calm and pay attention to cues for more affection seem to do well. Nudity, in particular, often arouses staff distress, yet professionals often display little regard for patients' privacy or modesty during baths or invasive procedures like enemas. Ongoing in-service training for staff and instruction for caregivers are recommended to increase understanding of, sensitivity to, and ability to deal calmly and tactfully with sexual behaviors and intimacy needs of Alzheimer patients.

SUMMARY

Nurses are on the frontline of responsibility and day-to-day service to Alzheimer patients. Their role demands that they be knowledgeable about and sensitive to a broad array of symptoms and methods of alleviation and management. Moreover, they must function within a situation for which there is no cure, but rather an inexorable downhill spiral. Often they must serve as instructor and interpreter to nonprofessional caregivers, usually family members who are upset at the progressive impairment of their loved one. Nurses are involved in support of families (Beam, 1984; Polk-Penrod, 1982; Rowe M, personal communication, 1985). Nurses function as liaisons between the patient, with whom they have direct daily contact, and doctors and other professionals, whose knowledge of the patient is less personal and concrete. Given this broad and difficult set of tasks, it is easy for the individual who is afflicted with Alzheimer's disease to get lost, to be seen as a conglomerate of symptoms and problems. And yet it is precisely the ability to establish and sustain a human, one-to-one relationship that lies at the core of good nursing care for Alzheimer patients. Alzheimer sufferers are above all human beings, and they need to be treated with kindness, attentiveness, and empathy. In caring for them our common humanity should be remembered, for none of us knows what the future holds for us.

3
Psychopharmacologic Interventions

Andrew Satlin and Jonathan O. Cole

Clinical and neurobiological research in Alzheimer's disease over the last decade suggests a complex pathology in this disorder. Pervasive intellectual impairment is a hallmark of Alzheimer's disease, but at various stages the disorder may cause personality change, impaired emotional responsiveness, anxiety and depression, and disturbances of motor functioning (see also Winograd, Chapter 1; Cohen, Chapter 5; Tune et al., Chapter 7). Abnormalities of cholinergic neurotransmission have been uniformly found in Alzheimer patients, and there is evidence that these may be a cause of the cognitive dysfunction. However, abnormalities of the dopaminergic, noradrenergic, serotonergic, gamma amino-butyric acid (GABAergic), and other neurotransmitter systems have also been detected in some patients, and the link between these disturbances and the clinical symptoms of Alzheimer's disease is not at all understood. By analogy with other medical disorders that have both a complex pathophysiology and a complex clinical presentation, such as diabetes mellitus, it would seem logical to presume an underlying etiology of Alzheimer's disease that triggers branching pathogenetic processes. Unfortunately, the etiology of Alzheimer's disease, which may have genetic, viral, toxic, or other components, is unknown. Once it is better understood, therapeutic strategies can be directed toward etiology, which will result not only in treatment of the disease, but perhaps in prevention as well.

With our current state of knowledge of this disease, rational pharmacologic approaches to Alzheimer's treatment are of two types.

Drugs are listed by both brand name and generic name in the Drug Index.

The first type attempts to treat the various psychiatric syndromes that are common in the clinical presentation of Alzheimer's disease. These include depression, psychosis with behavioral disturbance, anxiety, and sleep disorders.

The second approach involves research using drugs with the potential to correct the presumed neurochemical disturbances. Clinical success is measured by improvement in cognitive functioning. Most of these attempts have failed to produce clinically detectable improvement; so far they have minimal implications for the practicing clinician treating patients with Alzheimer's disease.

TREATMENT OF PSYCHIATRIC SYNDROMES IN ALZHEIMER'S DISEASE

Alzheimer patients may exhibit a variety of psychiatric syndromes in addition to deficits in memory and other intellectual functions. One recent study of 135 patients with Alzheimer's disease found that 7% had psychiatric symptoms or personality change as the initial presentation of the disease (Growdon, 1985). Many more patients develop such problems at one time or another in the course of their illness, though the proportion who do is unknown. Depression, anxiety, psychosis, disturbed behavior, and sleep disorders are among the most common manifestations. In many cases it is unclear whether these symptoms are manifestations of the underlying brain pathology, reactions to the loss of cognitive abilities, or a result of some combination of these two processes. Whatever the cause, psychiatric syndromes in Alzheimer patients often respond to psychotropic medication. Such treatment may be of dramatic benefit for patients suffering from Alzheimer's disease, as well as for their caregivers. The pharmacologic treatment of these psychiatric syndromes is reviewed below.

Depression

Much has been written about the syndrome of "pseudodementia" (Wells, 1979; McAllister, 1983; Shraberg, 1978; Grunhaus et al., 1983). This term has been coined to describe the clinical appearance of dementia in patients who do not have a progressive organic brain disease. Such patients do have a functional psychiatric illness, such as depression, and their dementia symptoms may resolve as the depression improves. Severe cognitive dysfunction can result from affective disorders, and this is seen most often in the elderly (McAllister, 1983). Nevertheless, an emphasis on distinguishing true dementia from the dementia syndrome of depression obscures the fact that depression and dementia often coexist in the same patient (see also Cohen, Chapter 5). Some authors believe that most patients who present with the dementia syndrome of depression (a term we prefer to pseudodementia) will be found to have persistent cognitive deficits even after their depression has been adequately treated (Reifler et al., 1982). Others disagree (La Rue, 1982), but definitive data are still lacking.

The coexistence of dementia and depression raises the question of whether dementing processes may trigger depression. This possibility is recognized in the DSM-III-R (American Psychiatric Association, 1987), which includes the diagnoses of "primary degenerative dementia of the Alzheimer type, senile onset, with depression and primary degenerative dementia of the Alzheimer type, presenile onset with depression." A biological basis for this association has not been proved, though a possible neurochemical relationship will be discussed below. However, dementia and depression may interact clinically. Many authors note that depression is common early in the course of Alzheimer's disease (Reifler et al., 1986; La Rue, 1982). It has been suggested that as patients become aware of declining cognitive abilities with resultant loss of independence, their self-esteem may be damaged, giving rise to a secondary depression. Symptoms include sadness, loss of energy, and withdrawal. These depressions are clinically similar to those seen in younger patients or nondemented elderly.

Later in the course of Alzheimer's disease, the relationship between dementia and depression may be more complex. Dementia may change the nature of depressive symptoms. In one report, an 80-year-old man with severe Alzheimer's disease developed agitation, psychosis, and bizarre behavior that responded to electroconvulsive therapy (ECT) (Demuth & Rand, 1980). The authors concluded that the elaboration and expression of typical depressive behavior, thoughts, and affect were hampered by impaired cognitive capacity and replaced by simpler equivalents. In cases such as this one, depression may be masked by the symptoms of dementia, which appear to predominate. Similarly, depression may worsen dementia. Shraberg (1978) described an 85-year-old man with dementia and a superimposed depression. On admission to the hospital he was disoriented and appeared a great deal more cognitively impaired than he had a month before. With treatment of his depression, improved cognition was noted clinically and documented by a slight improvement in IQ score, though some deficits due to dementia remained.

Reports such as the above suggest that as Alzheimer's disease progresses, potentially treatable depression may be harder to detect. In order not to miss treating these depressions, two criteria for suspecting them should be kept in mind while evaluating Alzheimer patients. First, any acute or rapid regression in behavior or functioning that cannot be explained by a new medical illness or environmental stress should suggest the possibility of depression. Second, any patient with Alzheimer's disease who develops psychosis or agitation and has a past history of affective illness, or a clear family history of affective illness, should also be considered for empirical antidepressant therapy.

The pharmacologic treatment of depression when it coexists with Alzheimer's disease rests on two considerations. First, most Alzheimer patients are elderly. Therefore, principles governing the use of antidepressant therapy in older persons must be applied. Second, neuronal damage resulting from Alzheimer's disease may alter the effects of antidepressant drug treatment. More research data are available for the former than for the latter.

Tricyclic antidepressants (TCAs) are the pharmacologic agents most frequently used in treating depression in all age groups. Since all the TCAs seem to be equally effective, the selection of an appropriate agent for a given patient is based on the different side-effect profiles of these drugs. In elderly patients, the most serious potential side effects fall into two classes: anticholinergic and cardiovascular.

Anticholinergic side effects include peripheral symptoms such as dry mouth, constipation, urinary retention, and blurry vision. These often exacerbate the slowed intestinal motility, urinary hesitancy due to prostatic hypertrophy, and poor vision due to cataracts and glaucoma that are common in the elderly (Salzman & van der Kolk, 1984). With higher doses of the TCAs, central nervous system toxicity may develop, presenting as delirium, with confusion, disorientation, agitation, and even hallucinations. The elderly seem to be more vulnerable than younger patients to a central anticholinergic toxic syndrome, so this side effect is to be especially avoided (Salzman, 1982). Demented elderly may be even more susceptible. A deficit in brain cholinergic function has been documented in Alzheimer patients (Bowen et al., 1976; Perry et al., 1978), and a recent study found that elderly patients with Alzheimer's disease were more sensitive than age-matched controls to the effects of the anticholinergic drug scopolamine on several tests of learning and memory (Sunderland et al., 1985). Data are not available on these effects with the therapeutic use of the TCAs in elderly Alzheimer patients, but a heightened anticholinergic sensitivity may be presumed with these drugs as well.

Memory loss associated with TCA use has been reported in some patients (Salzman & van der Kolk, 1984). This is probably a result of the anticholinergic properties of these drugs, though other mechanisms have been suggested (Cole et al., 1983). An important question is whether this side effect is more prominent in patients with Alzheimer's disease than in nondemented depressed elderly patients. If so, what implications does this have for pharmacologic treatment? There is little research to guide us in this area. One study found that amitriptyline, a TCA, resulted in a highly significant worsening of overall cognitive functioning in depressed patients who had some degree of cognitive dysfunction at baseline (Branconnier et al., 1981a). On the other hand, a prospective study of 46 elderly patients treated with TCAs found that only four developed confusional states, and none of 12 patients with evidence of mild to moderate dementia on baseline neuropsychological testing had drug-induced confusion (Meyers & Mei-Tal, 1983). One review concluded that confusional states directly caused by TCAs are not very frequent and do not seem increased in patients with dementia (Cole et al., 1983). There is a complex interaction of TCAs, depression, and dementia. Cognitive impairment from TCAs competes with cognitive improvement due to the relief of depression. Careful monitoring for possible effects on memory is, therefore, advisable when prescribing TCAs to patients with Alzheimer's disease.

Orthostatic hypotension is the most common cardiovascular side effect that can have serious consequences in elderly patients. Sudden drops in blood pressure may result in syncope and falling, stroke, or myocardial infarction. Research data are not available on orthostatic changes in individuals with Alzheimer's disease, so it is not known whether dementia increases the susceptibility to this side effect. Nortriptyline (Roose et al., 1981) and doxepin (Neshkes et al., 1985) may cause less orthostatic hypotension than the other TCAs, but there are not enough data to be definitive.

Sedation is another side effect that can be especially troublesome in the elderly. At times sedation may be desired, but in many patients sedative drugs lead to confusion and disorientation. Daytime drowsiness may also occur, which may exacerbate nighttime insomnia. Less sedating TCAs include desipramine and nortriptyline.

Aging also decreases the metabolism of most TCAs, leading to higher blood levels (Hicks et al., 1981). Thus TCAs should be prescribed in low starting doses. A good starting dose for nortriptyline is 10 mg a day, and for desipramine and doxepin, 25 mg a day. Increments of 10 mg of nortriptyline or 25 mg of desipramine or doxepin can be made every five to seven days. Response to nortriptyline may be seen at doses as low as 20 mg, and to desipramine and doxepin at 50 mg, although higher doses are often required. There is no information in the literature on the use of blood levels of antidepressant medication as a guide to therapy in patients who are both depressed and demented. Because full clinical effects may take four to six weeks, it is important not to abandon a therapeutic trial prematurely. On the other hand, some improvement should be manifested within the first week or two if data from non-demented can be extrapolated to demented depressed patients.

The neurochemistry of Alzheimer's disease suggests another intriguing approach to the pharmacotherapy of depression in this disease. Monoamine oxidase (MAO) enzyme activity is known to increase with age, and two groups found that platelet MAO activity is even higher in patients with dementia than in age-matched controls (Alexopoulos et al., 1984; Gottfries et al., 1983). This raises the interesting hypothesis that the MAO inhibitors (MAOIs) might be particularly suited for anti-depressant treatment of elderly patients with Alzheimer's disease. In one study, four out of nine patients without evidence of dementia, and all five with coexistent dementia and depression, had a significant remission of their depression on phenelzine or tranylcypromine, although they had failed to respond to other antidepressants (Ashford & Ford, 1979). Side effects were felt to be fewer and less persistent than with TCAs. Con-trolled clinical trials using MAOIs in depressed patients with Alzheimer's disease have not been done, but a recent report of two cases supports further investigation of this approach (Jenike, 1985). Another advantage is the low anticholinergic effect of the MAOIs, though they frequently cause dizziness and orthostatic hypotension. One drawback to the use of these drugs in demented patients is the need to avoid foods with a high tyramine content, which can interact with the MAOIs to cause a hypertensive crisis. Patients with memory impairment should be in a supervised setting to minimize the risk of precipitating such a reaction if MAOIs are to be used. If adequate dietary monitoring can be assured, a trial with an MAOI is certainly warranted in patients with Alzheimer's disease and depression. Phenelzine may be prescribed starting at 15 mg a day, with the dose increased by 15 mg every few days, until 80% MAO inhibition has been achieved. This measure has been found to correlate well with therapeutic efficacy in a group of elderly patients without dementia (Georgotas et al., 1983), although no data are available in the demented depressed.

Trazodone, a nontricyclic antidepressant, can also be considered for these patients. It is devoid of anticholinergic properties and does not cause constipation, though its alpha-adrenergic side effects can produce dry mouth. This side effect is often incorrectly considered an anti-cholinergic effect. Confusion was noted in two of 19 patients on trazo-done in the only double-blind, placebo-controlled trial in elderly de-pressed patients, although therapeutic efficacy was equivalent to that of imipramine, and overall side effects were fewer (Gerner et al., 1980). No reports exist of controlled clinical trials using trazodone in demented depressed patients. Some clinicians are enthusiastic about the drug in this population, while others find the sedative side effects disabling. The starting dose should be as low as possible. Unfortunately, the lowest-dose single pill is 50 mg, but it can be broken in half to start treatment at 25 mg a day.

Electroconvulsive therapy (ECT) is another effective and safe treatment for the demented depressed elderly patient (Salzman, 1982). It is not known whether ECT has differential effects on depression in patients with coexistent Alzheimer's disease, compared to nondemented subjects. However, ECT may be the treatment of choice in psychotic depression, and patients with coexistent depression and Alzheimer's disease often exhibit psychosis as part of their clinical syndrome. Four such cases in the literature, reported by three groups, all responded dramatically to ECT (Demuth & Rand, 1980; McAllister & Price, 1983; Snow & Wells, 1981). Cognitive impairment improved in two of these patients and was unchanged in two others. For patients with psychotic depression superimposed on Alzheimer's disease, or for those patients who cannot tolerate the side effects of antidepressant medication, ECT is a valuable therapeutic alternative, despite the lack of controlled studies.

Psychoses and Behavioral Disturbances

Psychoses and severe disturbances of behavior overlap clinically in the elderly Alzheimer patient and will be discussed together in this section. Alzheimer's disease may itself cause psychotic symptoms and behavioral disturbances, but a biochemical basis for these effects is not known. It is reasonable to expect that as cognitive skills become impaired, resulting in decreased ability to accurately perceive and interpret reality, behavior will become unpredictable and inappropriate, and thinking will become illogical. Paranoia, fearfulness, agitation, irascibility, wandering, restlessness, assaultiveness, and inappropriate social behavior accompany the deterioration of basic intellectual functions in many, though not all, demented patients. These symptoms may become major problems in the management of patients with Alzheimer's disease, whether at home, in hospitals, or in nursing homes. Two general classes of drugs, the neuroleptics and the benzodiazepines, are frequently used as symptomatic treatments.

Neuroleptics

Neuroleptic medication is the mainstay of treatment for agitation and anxiety in dementia (Shader & Greenblatt, 1982). A survey of 12 VA hospitals (Prien et al., 1975) found that among 1,276 elderly psychiatric patients, the most frequently prescribed drugs were the antipsychotic agents, which were given to 44% of the total and 36% of the demented. Unfortunately, the efficacy of neuroleptic medication in demented patients with behavioral disturbance has not been firmly demonstrated. Among seven placebo-controlled trials performed before 1980, three found clear benefit of neuroleptic medication (Hamilton & Bennett, 1962a; Sugerman et al., 1964; Seager, 1955) but four found limited or no benefit (Abse & Dahlstrom, 1960; Barton & Hurst, 1966; Hamilton & Bennett, 1962b; Rada & Kellner, 1976). These studies are difficult to interpret because some included patients with psychiatric diagnoses other than dementia, and they are difficult to compare because the studies did not use the same outcome measures.

Two placebo-controlled studies of neuroleptic medication in more rigorously diagnosed patient groups offer more clues about the appropriate use of these drugs. Loxapine and haloperidol, when compared to placebo in 61 hospitalized geriatric patients with dementia, both yielded improvement in suspiciousness, hallucinatory behavior, excitement, unsociability, and uncooperativeness (Petrie et al., 1982). Overall, marked or moderate improvement was seen in about a third of patients who received an active drug, compared to 9% who received a placebo. Another study found roughly the same rate of overall improvement among demented patients treated with either loxapine or thioridazine, but the degree of change was not significantly different from placebo (Barnes et al., 1982). On individual symptoms, only loxapine resulted in significant improvement compared to placebo; anxiety, excitement, emotional lability, and uncooperativeness were reduced. Patients most likely to benefit were those with the most severe behavioral symptoms at baseline.

Both of these studies reported a high incidence of adverse effects, ranging from 33% to 90%. Sedation, extrapyramidal effects, and orthostatic hypotension were the most common, each occurring in about 25% to 50% of all subjects in both series.

Alzheimer's disease was the diagnosis in over half of the patients in both studies, with the remainder mostly diagnosed as multiinfarct dementia. When analyzed separately, there was no relationship between diagnosis and treatment efficacy (Barnes et al., 1982).

Taken together, these two studies do not offer a great deal of encouragement for the use of neuroleptics in patients with Alzheimer's disease and behavioral disturbance. While one in three patients improved, more than one in 10 got worse. Side effects were common and may have accounted for some of the clinical worsening.

Another consideration when prescribing neuroleptics is the risk of tardive dyskinesia (TD). This disorder, characterized by involuntary movement of the tongue, lips, and face, is associated with the long-term use of neuroleptic medication and has an increased incidence in the elderly (Smith & Baldessarini, 1980). In addition, dementia may contribute to the development of dyskinesias. Several studies reported high prevalence of spontaneous dyskinesia among samples that included patients with varying degrees of dementia (Blowers, 1981; Bourgeois et al., 1980; Delwaide & Desseilles, 1977). Conversely, two other studies found increased incidence of organic brain disorders in patients with TD, compared to controls (Edwards, 1970; Itil et al., 1981). Thus elderly Alzheimer patients may represent an especially high risk group for the development of TD, compromising further the potential usefulness of neuroleptics in this population.

Nevertheless, for Alzheimer patients with paranoid ideation, hallucinations, excitement, emotional lability, and uncooperativeness, especially if the symptoms are severe, the studies cited above suggest that neuroleptics may be beneficial, and we know of no better drug available at this time. The choice of an appropriate agent in a particular patient should be based on avoiding the side effects that that patient would tolerate least. In general, neuroleptics with higher milligram potency have greater extrapyramidal, but fewer anticholinergic, side effects. Drugs of this type include haloperidol. By contrast, thioridazine, a low-potency drug, causes more sedation, hypotension, and anticholinergic effects, but fewer extrapyramidal reactions. Sometimes a drug of intermediate potency, such as acetophenazine or perphenazine, may have the fewest undesirable side effects. Whatever medication is tried first, intolerable side effects dictate change to a drug with a different side-effect profile.

As with all other psychotropic medications, low doses of neuroleptics are recommended. Appropriate starting daily doses are 0.5 to 1.0 mg for haloperidol, 2 to 4 mg for perphenazine, and 10 to 25 mg for thioridazine. The dose is then gradually increased or decreased depending on the clinical results or side effects. Several weeks may be required for maximal response. Target symptoms should be clearly defined for a given patient before medication is begun. Then, if improvement is not clearly seen in these symptoms after several weeks, a drug of a different class should be tried.

Benzodiazepines

Benzodiazepines have also been recommended for the treatment of agitation in dementia. Several early controlled trials indicate that benzodiazepines are more effective than placebo in controlling behavioral symptoms in demented patients (Beber, 1965; Chesrow et al., 1965; Sanders,

1965), but published studies comparing a neuroleptic and a benzo-diazepine in geriatric patients are rare. Three investigators compared thioridazine to diazepam. One reported reductions in agitation, anxious mood, and fearfulness with thioridazine (Covington, 1975); another found greater improvement in anxiety, fearfulness, and overall mental illness with thioridazine, but more improvement in agitation, insomnia, and intellect with diazepam (Kirven & Montero, 1973). The third, and only placebo-controlled comparison, found improvement with both drugs (Stotsky, 1984) but a significantly greater change in a majority of measures in the patients on thioridazine. Insomnia was the only symptom for which diazepam was more effective. In another investigation, oxaze-pam was found superior to both thioridazine and haloperidol in control-ling agitation and restlessness in elderly demented patients when these medications were tried sequentially (Tewfik et al., 1970).

The available literature is thus inconclusive about the relative effica-cy and symptom specificity of neuroleptics and benzodiazepines in Alzheimer's disease. Side effects of the benzodiazepines (see section be-low on "Anxiety") mandate caution in their use with elderly demented patients and argue in favor of relatively short- rather than long-acting agents. Very short-acting drugs are best avoided because of their high peak blood levels. We would recommend a trial of a benzodiazepine in the behaviorally disturbed Alzheimer patient who meets the following criteria: (1) paranoia, hallucinations, or other overt symptoms of psy-chosis are not present; (2) insomnia is present; (3) neuroleptics are ineffective or produce unmanageable side effects. More will be said about the use of benzodiazepines in Alzheimer's disease in the sections below on "Anxiety" and "Sleep Disorders."

Lithium

The role of lithium in the treatment of psychosis and behavioral dis-turbance in Alzheimer's disease is controversial. Case reports describing improvement with lithium have generally involved patients with organic brain syndromes caused not by Alzheimer's disease but by other pathologic processes. In one series of 10 patients, six had a clearly positive response, but five of these suffered from alcoholism and all had symptoms of depression (Williams & Goldstein, 1979). The only patient with Alzheimer's disease in this group was one of the two nonresponders. Another report described an Alzheimer patient who had decreased agita-tion, hostility, and wandering when treated with lithium but noted that the patient also had symptoms resembling mania (Havens & Cole, 1982).

Alzheimer's disease also appears to adversely modulate the effect of lithium on the brain. In Alzheimer patients, severe neurotoxicity may develop to lithium at lower levels than in patients without dementia (Strayhorn & Nash, 1977). Neurological illness of any sort has been associated with poor treatment response to lithium in elderly patients with bipolar disorder and with the development of neurotoxicity (Himmelhoch et al., 1980). In another report (Kelwala et al., 1984), five of six patients with Alzheimer's disease who had extrapyramidal symptoms prior to lithium treatment developed worsening of these symptoms, as well as worsened cognitive function.

These complex and potentially harmful interactions of Alzheimer's disease, lithium, and possibly extrapyramidal symptoms, together with very limited evidence of benefit, limit the indications for this medication in Alzheimer's disease. We recommend its use only in those patients who have a past history of bipolar disorder or alcoholism, or in whom the clinical presentation is similar to mania, or for whom past response to lithium has been documented. We would be especially cautious in prescribing lithium to Alzheimer patients who also have parkinsonian symptoms or other evidence of extrapyramidal dysfunction.

Anxiety

Anxiety, like depression, may have different presentations and treatment requirements at different times in the progression of Alzheimer's disease. Early in the course of the illness, anxiety is an understandable reaction to the realization of cognitive decline and the anticipation of increasing loss of intellect. Often anxiety and depression are indistinguishable at this point. With progression of the dementia, and decreased awareness of its effects, the symptoms of anxiety often become less prominent, but the agitation and behavioral problems that replace them may in fact be manifestations of anxiety. Pacing, restlessness, irritability, and even aggression and assaultiveness may occur.

Anxiety in the early stages of Alzheimer's disease may not require pharmacologic intervention. Often anxiety is due to realistic concerns about lack of adequate support from others or of financial resources. Provision of additional social support may be enough to alleviate the anxiety. Psychotherapeutic and social service interventions may be effective at this early stage (see also Cohen, Chapter 5; Brody, Chapter 6; Tune et al., Chapter 7; Sainer, Chapter 11).

Clinical experience suggests that anxiety often coexists with depression in early stages of Alzheimer's disease. If depression is suspected and pharmacological remedies are required, antidepressant medication should be tried before antianxiety drugs are prescribed.

No controlled studies have been published on drug therapy for demented patients with anxiety. Benzodiazepines are most commonly prescribed, though side effects of these medications in the elderly include excess sedation, confusion, disinhibition with paradoxical agitation, unsteady gait, dysarthria, and uncoordination (Shader & Greenblatt, 1982). Clinical experience suggests that these toxicities are more common with increased duration of treatment, and we recommend weekly reassessment of the need for medication.

Benzodiazepines such as oxazepam, with short half-lives and without active metabolites, accumulate to a lesser degree and are eliminated more rapidly after treatment is discontinued than benzodiazepines such as diazepam, with long half-lives and active metabolites (Salzman et al., 1983). On the other hand, short half-lives mean that the drug must be given in multiple daily doses, which may reduce compliance in patients with memory impairment, resulting in decreased clinical effectiveness. As with other psychotropic drugs, decreased drug metabolism and increased sensitivity of the aging brain to drug effects dictate the use of low doses of medication. Oxazepam should be started at a dose of 10 mg two to three times a day, and the total daily dose should not exceed 60 mg.

In patients with advanced cognitive impairment, the benzodiazepines may cause increased confusion, disinhibition, and agitation (Salzman, 1984). For Alzheimer patients, low doses of a neuroleptic drug, as discussed in the previous section, may be preferable. Sedation is apt to be an undesirable side effect in these patients, since it may exacerbate confusion, which can result in greater irritability and anxiety. A high-potency neuroleptic such as haloperidol is low in sedative effects.

Sleep Disturbances

The pharmacologic treatment of sleep disorders in Alzheimer's disease is based on the same general principles as the treatment of anxiety, except that even greater caution must be exercised because of the effects of Alzheimer's disease on sleep patterns. With normal aging, the stages of sleep change (Kales & Kales, 1974). As a result, older persons tend to spend more hours in bed, although actual time spent asleep declines. It takes older persons longer to fall asleep, and they experience more frequent awakenings through the night. This fragmentation of the normal sleep–wake cycle is exacerbated by the pathologic changes in Alzheimer's disease (Prinz et al., 1982a). With cognitive decline and weakening of the internal biological clock, the patient may nap more frequently during the day and be unable to sleep for long periods at night. Hypnotic medications, though often effective inducers of sleep, do not improve the fragmented sleep patterns. Use of these drugs may exacerbate confusion and sedation during waking periods, further compromising overall cognitive functioning.

Research data are not available regarding the pharmacologic treatment of insomnia in demented patients. The benzodiazepines are used widely for nighttime sleeplessness. However, they may lose their hypnotic effect after 20 to 30 days of continual use (Regestein, 1984) and therefore should not be prescribed for longer than a month. Use after this period may only serve to prevent increased insomnia resulting from drug withdrawal and can lead to psychological dependence.

As discussed earlier, drugs with short half-lives and without active metabolites, such as oxazepam, are preferable to flurazepam or diazepam. Even drugs with short half-lives, however, may produce mild daytime sedation with more than two weeks of repeated daily dosing (Salzman et al., 1983). In addition, intermediate-acting benzodiazepines such as oxazepam and temazepam have been associated with the development of early-morning insomnia after one to two weeks of continual use (Kales et al., 1983) and with significant rebound insomnia after abrupt withdrawal (Regestein, 1984). These are further reasons for limiting the duration of pharmacotherapy for insomnia. Without research data on effective doses in demented patients, our recommendations are based on clinical experience: initial hypnotic doses are 10 to 20 mg of oxazepam, 15 to 30 mg of temazepam, and 0.25 to 0.5 mg of lorazepam.

In some Alzheimer patients, neuroleptic medication may be preferable to the benzodiazepines for sleep disturbance, though no controlled studies of this population are available. One study of 20 nondemented elderly patients found that 25 mg of thioridazine produced longer sleep at night, with less daytime drowsiness, than 10 mg of nitrazepam, a benzodiazepine (Linnoila & Viukari, 1976). However, in many cases the neuroleptics will also have prolonged effects, leading to sleep during the day. As with the benzodiazepines, tolerance to their sedating effects may develop after two to three weeks (Regestein, 1984). In general, any medication with the potential for exacerbating confusion should be employed very judiciously with the Alzheimer patient, and the value of its continued use should be regularly reassessed (see also Winograd, Chapter 1).

APPROACHES BASED ON
PRESUMED BRAIN ABNORMALITIES

Overview

Over the years, a variety of drug treatments has been suggested for Alzheimer's disease based on prevailing theories about the biology of the disorder. In most cases, enthusiasm based on early reports has become tempered by mixed results in open trials, and eventually negative conclusions have emerged from double-blind, placebo-controlled experiments.

In reviewing this large body of research, attempts to draw conclusions are hampered by methodological problems in the studies themselves. Not long ago, most cases of dementia were considered to have a vascular etiology, and most treatment strategies were based on this theory. Earlier therapeutic investigations are also difficult to interpret because they included patients with Alzheimer's disease, multiinfarct dementia (MID), and other dementing disorders in unknown proportions. More recent studies have altered our conceptions about the epidemiology of dementia. Alzheimer's disease is now believed to cause roughly half of all cases of clinical dementia, with MID responsible for about 15% and some combination of the two for another 20% (Raskin DE, 1985). Recent therapeutic investigations have, therefore, employed rigorous criteria to select subjects with probable Alzheimer's disease, which is the most precise diagnosis that can be made without biopsy or autopsy confirmation.

Even with clearly defined patient populations, other methodological problems have made pharmacologic studies in Alzheimer's disease difficult to perform and interpret. First, the need for accurate diagnosis generally makes the inclusion of patients with mild Alzheimer's disease impossible, since no biologic marker exists for this condition. Many treatment studies with negative outcomes may be biased by the use of patients with moderate or severe disease, in whom neuronal loss may have markedly limited treatment response.

Second, neuropsychological tests and behavioral measures for assessing changes with drug treatment have not been standardized. Different tests may be needed in order to detect change at different levels of impairment. Also, studies may easily err on the side of too few measures, which may miss unexpected findings, or too many, which may result in positive findings not achieving statistical significance (see also LaRue, Chapter 12).

A third problem is that many drugs with possible salutary effects in Alzheimer's disease may have narrow therapeutic dose ranges, and these may vary widely among individuals. This will be discussed in the section on neurotransmitters, but sufficient attention has not been paid to this possibility in trials with other drugs.

Finally, symptoms in Alzheimer's disease represent a complex interaction of psychosocial, environmental, and general medical conditions together with brain pathology. These variables make evaluation of drug effects difficult.

Before describing the drugs that have been tested, a word about their classification is in order. Our knowledge about the neurochemical and physiologic abnormalities in Alzheimer's disease has expanded dramatically over the last few years. One might expect that therapies originally proposed and tested on the basis of theories that are no longer accepted would now be obsolete. Paradoxically this is not always the case. A good example is dihydroergotoxine. Originally, this drug was believed to be a vasodilator, and its use was based on the theory that cerebrovascular insufficiency was the major cause of dementia. While this theory is no longer accepted, dihydroergotoxine has been found to improve brain electrical activity by increasing the activity of enzymes of intermediary glucose metabolism under some conditions (Meier-Ruge et al., 1975), and it is now considered one of the "metabolic enhancers." The classification of drugs into the groups listed below, therefore, is largely arbitrary. It is worth noting, however, that as our knowledge about the properties of these drugs increases, we become better able to understand the pathology of the Alzheimer's disease process itself.

Psychostimulants

Alzheimer patients often appear apathetic and withdrawn, with impaired mental alertness and decreased physical energy. Stimulant treatment would appear to make clinical sense, and a number of different agents have been tried. Among these are methylphenidate and magnesium pemoline. According to one review (Ferris, 1981), none of three controlled trials of methylphenidate found any effect on cognitive functioning, though one (Branconnier & Cole, 1980) found improvement in mood, particularly for patients with greater levels of initial depression. Magnesium pemoline is another amphetamine-like stimulant with some positive effects on memory in animal studies but with consistently negative results in controlled clinical trials (Ferris, 1981). Other drugs with stimulant properties, including pentylenetetrazol and pipradrol, have been equally disappointing (Cole, 1980). As with methylphenidate, any improvement seen tends to be in overall behavior or mood, rather than in cognitive performance.

Numerous claims have been made for the efficacy in dementia of a 2% procaine hydrochloride solution. A review of the literature on this agent concluded that there is no evidence that it has any value in the treatment of disease in older patients, except perhaps for a mild antidepressant effect (Ostfeld et al., 1977); and a controlled, double-blind study failed to confirm any efficacy as an antidepressant (Olsen et al., 1978).

Vasodilators and Metabolic Enhancers

Drugs that have been classified by different authors as vasodilators or metabolic enhancers will be treated as a group here. Although many such drugs have been extensively studied, their mechanism of action is still not clear. Several, such as dihydroergotoxine, papaverine, and naftidrofuryl, which were first studied for their putative ability to dilate cerebral blood vessels, have been found to have other effects on cellular metabolism and neurotransmission. Many attractive theories have been presented to explain the relevance of these actions to the treatment of dementia. In fact, a variety of these drugs have been found to have slight, though definite, benefit in selected patients (Yesavage et al., 1979). However, the relationship between the known pharmacologic properties of these agents and their clinical efficacy is not yet established. It is possible that additional actions of these drugs may be discovered, or that newer vasodilators may also be found to enhance metabolism or even to have unique effects in the demented brain.

Dihydroergotoxine

Dihydroergotoxine is a combination of three dihydrogenated ergot alkaloids. It is the most widely prescribed and studied cerebral metabolic enhancer. Animal experiments have found that dihydroergotoxine protects against impaired glucose metabolism induced by hypothermia and ischemia. It also may act as an alpha-adrenergic antagonist and as a serotonin and dopamine agonist (Hollister & Yesavage, 1984). Any of these actions may theoretically be useful in the treatment of Alzheimer's disease. Abnormalities of the cholinergic neurotransmitter system have been regularly noted in brain tissue from Alzheimer patients, and studies suggest that impaired cerebral carbohydrate oxidation results in proportional decreases in the synthesis of acetylcholine (ACh) (Gibson GE et al., 1978). Thus the observed deficits in the synthesis of ACh in the brains of patients with Alzheimer's disease may be secondary to a metabolic deficiency (Reisberg, 1981), and treatments such as dihydroergotoxine that attempt to correct these deficits may be successful. Abnormalities of other neurotransmitter systems possibly affected by dihydroergotoxine will be discussed in more detail below in the section on "Neurotransmitters."

There have been a number of reviews of studies using dihydroergotoxine. In one review, improvement was considered to be of practical importance in 18 of 22 studies, or 80%, but there was no consensus regarding which symptoms were most likely to improve (Yesavage et al., 1979). In a recent study, dihydroergotoxine was found to be significantly better than placebo, but no changes were observed in either group on quantitative psychometric test results (van Loveren-Huyben et al., 1984). Numerous studies in the aggregate demonstrate slight statistical advantage for dihydroergotoxine over placebo, but do not document meaningful clinical improvement in cognition.

Other Vasodilators

Naftidrofuryl, a vasodilator also said to act as a metabolic enhancer (Fontaine et al., 1968), is reported to have had practical benefit in seven well-designed studies, and even appeared to improve cognition in some studies (Yesavage et al., 1979). However, another review concluded that the drug has not been shown to improve blind clinical ratings, despite small improvements on neuropsychological tests (Branconnier, 1983).

Papaverine, another vasodilator, has done consistently worse than Hydergine in all five reported studies (Crook, 1985). Several other drugs with vasodilator properties, including cyclandelate, isoxsuprine, vincamine, nylidrin hydrochloride and cinnarizine, have been found to have limited, if any, efficacy (Yesavage et al., 1979). It is interesting that none of these drugs has been postulated to have metabolic effects other than the ability to dilate blood vessels. Yesavage has noted that only six of 22 studies with drugs of this type claim practical benefit, compared to 27 of 31 trials of vasodilators with other enhancing effects on metabolism. This is not surprising, in light of evidence that reduced cerebral blood flow is the result, not the cause, of cerebral atrophy (Obrist, 1972) and that vasodilator therapy may actually reduce blood flow to ischemic areas (Cook & James, 1981).

Nootropics

The term "nootropic" has been coined to refer to drugs which are presumed to enhance integrative brain function (Giurgea, 1979). The prototype of this class is piracetam, and newer related compounds include oxiracetam, etiracetam, pramiracetam, and aniracetam. These drugs are reportedly devoid of toxic effects (Itil, 1983) and appear to function as metabolic enhancers. Piracetam has been found to increase brain levels of adenosine triphosphate (ATP) (Gobert, 1972), though it has also been proposed that these agents may act as neurotransmitters (Wurtman, 1985b). Administration of piracetam to rats reduces hippocampal ACh levels, suggesting that it increases the firing rate of presynaptic cholinergic neurons. Wurtman hypothesizes that the drug may assume, within the brain, a conformation resembling an excitatory transmitter for which receptors exist on cholinergic neurons. This would explain preliminary findings, in both animals and humans, that piracetam in combination with ACh precursors has a memory-enhancing effect markedly greater than that of either compound alone (Bartus et al., 1981; Smith RC et al., 1984).

Studies of piracetam and the other nootropics include a large number of uncontrolled trials with positive results, but controlled clinical studies in Alzheimer's disease have been equivocal (Ferris, 1981). Preliminary observations of the newer homologues suggest some efficacy (Itil et al., 1982; Mizuki et al., 1984) but also indicate the need for testing a wide range of doses.

Neuropeptides

Neuropeptides have been the subject of much research in the treatment of Alzheimer's disease. These protein fragments are often structurally related to peripheral hormones, in some cases being parts of longer hormone chains. They are produced and active in the central nervous system (CNS) and may function directly as neurotransmitters or have other modulating roles in neuronal metabolism or neurotransmission. Neuropeptides related to adrenocorticotropic hormone (ACTH) and others similar to vasopressin (VP) have been most studied. They have been postulated to function as neurotransmitters, or to facilitate neurotransmission, in a variety of neural systems in the tracts among the hypothalamus, septum, and hippocampus (Wurtman, 1985b; Goodnick & Gershon, 1984). These are areas believed to be involved in the formation of memory.

A large body of animal data suggests that several peptides related to ACTH and VP affect performance on a variety of memory tests. These animal studies, and the clinical investigations to which they have led, have been reviewed in detail elsewhere (Tinklenberg & Thornton, 1983). The reviewers concluded that both animal and human studies with neuropeptides reveal definite effects on behavior in certain conditions. However, these effects do not seem to be on intrinsic memory formation, but rather on memory modulating processes or nonspecific factors that affect task performance, such as arousal or attention. As a treatment for Alzheimer's disease, most well-designed trials have been negative (Tinklenberg & Thornton, 1983). The most consistent effects can again be explained as nonspecific CNS stimulation with secondary changes in attention or mood. In this respect both ACTH and VP neuropeptides may function much as several of the other classes of drugs described above. More recent work has tended to confirm these conclusions (Soininen et al., 1985; Martin et al., 1983; Reding & DiPonte, 1983; Peabody et al., 1985).

Interventions in other neurohumoral systems have also been proposed as possible treatment for Alzheimer patients. Studies have suggested a role of endogenous opioid systems in learning, possibly related to modulation of a variety of other neurotransmitter systems, particularly the gamma-aminobutyric acid (GABA) system (Reisberg et al., 1983b). On this basis, several trials of naloxone, an opioid antagonist, have been conducted. While an early report was positive (Reisberg et al., 1983a), the results were not replicated in a subsequent open trial (Blass et al., 1983) or a double-blind, placebo-controlled trial (Tariot et al., 1985).

Neurotransmitters

Several lines of evidence suggest that abnormalities of cholinergic neurotransmitter systems in the brain may be a primary cause of memory impairment in Alzheimer's disease. Studies of postmortem brain tissue of Alzheimer patients have revealed a deficiency of the enzyme choline acetyltransferase (CAT), which is needed for the synthesis of acetylcholine (ACh) (Bowen et al., 1976; Davies & Maloney, 1976). Furthermore, this deficiency is most marked in those brain areas where the concentrations of neurofibrillary tangles and neuritic plaques are greatest (Bartus et al., 1982) and is proportional both to plaque number and to severity of dementia (Perry et al., 1978). Most cholinergic input to the cerebral cortex originates in the nucleus basalis of Meynert, where a loss of up to 80% of neurons has been found in Alzheimer's disease (Whitehouse et al., 1981). Finally, disturbances in cholinergic neurotransmission produced in young normal subjects by the administration of anticholinergic drugs such as scopolamine result in memory deficits similar to those seen in Alzheimer patients (Drachman & Leavitt, 1974). A recent study extending these findings to patients with Alzheimer's disease found that subjects were more sensitive than controls to the effects of scopolamine on cognitive measures (Sunderland et al., 1985). This evidence, together with that from studies suggesting that postsynaptic muscarinic cholinergic receptors are not affected in Alzheimer's disease (Davies & Verth, 1977; Reisine et al., 1978), has been the stimulus for a variety of strategies to treat Alzheimer's disease by enhancing cholinergic neurotransmission. Three basic approaches have been tested: ACh precursor loading, anticholinesterases to limit ACh breakdown, and postsynaptic agents to directly stimulate ACh receptors.

Generally, most studies of ACh precursors have used either choline or lecithin, and most well-designed studies with both of these substances have not been effective (Goodnick & Gershon, 1984). More recent studies, however, utilizing higher doses and longer treatment durations, have been a bit more encouraging. One study using a preparation containing at least 90% phosphatidylcholine in doses up to 25 gm a day for six months found improvement in some psychometric measures at the end of the test period, though not at further six-month follow-up (Levy et al., 1983). Another study using the best dose among 10 gm, 15 gm, and 20 gm of lecithin as determined for individual patients in a preliminary experiment found no significant improvement over six months, but there was some evidence that the lecithin treatment may have decreased the rate of progression of the disease in 12 of 13 patients (Weintraub et al., 1983). Complex and unpredicted effects were found in a third study using high dose, long-term lecithin treatment, with improvement occurring only in a subgroup of relatively poor compliers (Little et al., 1985). The authors suggest that older patients, who were more likely to be poor compliers, might be more likely to have a pure cholinergic deficit.

While precursors alone have not been impressive in the treatment of Alzheimer's disease, it is possible that precursor pretreatment may be of greater use when agents that increase the firing rates of presynaptic neurons are administered simultaneously (Johns et al., 1983). As already noted, piracetam may have this effect. One study using a combination of piracetam and lecithin suggested a greater alleviation of selective memory deficits with these two agents together than with lecithin alone (Smith RC et al., 1984). However, this additive effect has not yet been confirmed.

Trials with the anticholinesterases physostigmine and tetrahydroaminoacridine (THA) have generally been more encouraging, especially when "best doses" were first determined for each individual and when testing measures were chosen to maximize the chance of detecting change (Johns et al., 1983). For such treatment to be useful clinically, oral agents with longer half-lives and fewer peripheral side effects will need to be tested. Two studies of oral physostigmine failed to demonstrate improvement (Jotkowitz, 1983; Caltagirone et al., 1982); this drug has had slight benefit when given in combination with oral lecithin (Levin & Peters, 1984; Thal et al., 1983; Weintraub et al., 1983). THA has a longer half-life than oral physostigmine and has fewer peripheral side effects, but this agent has not been extensively studied. One uncontrolled trial employing parenteral THA found significant memory improvement in some subjects (Summers et al., 1981), but a study of oral THA in combination with lecithin had more equivocal results (Kaye et al., 1982). A recent enthusiastic report of oral THA has inspired efforts to conduct replication studies to look for efficacy with this approach (Summers et al., 1986).

Investigations of postsynaptic cholinergic receptor agonists are still very preliminary. Slight improvement with arecoline, comparable in degree to that achieved with physostigmine, was found in one study (Christie et al., 1981), but arecoline has significant toxicity. A newer agent, RS86, appears to be better tolerated than arecoline, and beneficial effects on cognitive function, mood, and social behavior were found in preliminary trials with this drug (Wettstein & Spiegel, 1984). In most such studies, only a minority of patients have been found to improve clinically.

An interesting new approach is the infusion of a muscarinic agonist, bethanechol chloride, directly into the cerebrospinal fluid of Alzheimer patients using an implantable system (Harbaugh et al., 1984). Positive subjective responses have been reported in a few patients, while complications have been worrisome in others. The treatment is invasive and potentially hazardous, but if it leads to substantial improvement in some patients, such patients should be identified.

CONCLUSION

Despite extensive investigations, it is clear that a satisfactory pharmacologic treatment for Alzheimer's disease has not yet been found, although identifiable psychiatric syndromes complicating the dementia can often be treated symptomatically. Effective pharmacologic treatment for Alzheimer's disease will only be achieved by extensive basic and clinical research. As more is learned about the biochemical and neuropathologic processes in this disorder, novel approaches based on these discoveries may hold promise. Clinicians and other caregivers should keep abreast of current research in which their patients might participate. Information may be obtained from local chapters of the Alzheimer's Disease and Related Disorders Association (ADRDA), a national organization whose goal is to promote awareness, research, and treatment of Alzheimer's disease and related disorders. Through the combined efforts of researchers, patients, and other concerned individuals, better drug therapies for Alzheimer's disease should soon be found.

Supported in part by grant I KO8 AG-00236-01 from the National Institute on Aging, to Dr. Satlin. The authors wish to thank Elaine Beroz and Karen-Lee Rosenthal for their preparation of the manuscript.

4

Ethical Considerations

Christine K. Cassel and Mary Kane Goldstein

Modern medical science has developed technological capabilities to prolong life beyond all previous expectations. It has also created complex structures of health care, involving coordination of vast systems of information and the expertise and authority of diverse professionals. Technological options and expanded presumption of individual rights raise complicated legal as well as ethical questions for medical practice concerning treatment choice and informed consent.

Nowhere are the ethical dilemmas created by technological advances and shifts in social attitude more pressing than in the care of people suffering from Alzheimer's disease. Work with Alzheimer patients entails all of the ethical issues common to working with other sick persons, as well as those unique to this specific condition. The severity of the disease and the growing numbers of people afflicted, combined with our enhanced ability to prolong life, make systematic understanding of ethical choices a matter of prime concern. This chapter will discuss the principles of biomedical ethics; practical approaches to the ethical dilemmas; the health professional as ethicist; ethical dilemmas in Alzheimer's disease; and future concerns. This chapter is *not* intended, and cannot be, a guide to avoidance of legal entanglement. We recognize that in an individual instance, the health care provider may feel ethically compelled toward a stance that is not supported by law. Given our culture, diverse moral heritage, and the complexity of new questions introduced by advanced technology, the law is at some times self-contradictory, at other times silent, and in no case a substitute for individual ethical decision making. Because the law is also a guide to the considered opinion of careful thinkers, legal cases will in some instances be cited for illustrative purposes.

THE PRINCIPLES OF BIOMEDICAL ETHICS

The principles of ethical action are shaped to one's cultural context within the tradition of Western culture. Traditions of Judaism, Christianity, secular, political, and social philosophy all contribute somewhat different perspectives (Jonsen, 1982). There is, however, a remarkably broad commonality among them. Scholars looking at ethical problems in medicine over the last two decades have established a framework based largely on three fundamental principles: respect for persons, beneficence, and justice.

Respect for Persons

This is a principle on which our legal system of rights and constitutional entitlements is based. It operates to insure harmonious interactions in the human community. In medical care, it has major implications for disclosure of information, informed consent, and self-determination. One should, in most cases, be frank with patients about their diagnosis, about what is known and not known about that diagnosis, and enlist them as partners when decision making of any ambiguous nature needs to be done. The exceptions to this are the few instances in which it seems medically or psychiatrically dangerous to give the information to the patient or, as sometimes happens, when the patient requests not to be told, asking that the doctor make all decisions for him or her. It becomes difficult in cases of cognitive disorder or in aphasia, where it is difficult to know how much the patient understands. Still, the effort must be made, and it is often surprising how much is understood in either case. With patients who have memory deficits, one must be prepared to repeat the information patiently, sometimes many times over. Informed consent is often an ongoing process of communication rather than a single encounter focused on the signing of a piece of paper.

Another aspect of respect is self-determination, also referred to as "patient autonomy." This principle demands that patients be allowed to decide the most favorable courses for themselves, according to their own value systems. It is a common pitfall for health professionals to judge patients' decisions by their own value systems rather than the patients'. Classically, we explain that a patient is making a wrong decision because he or she does not understand enough or does not have the medical knowledge that we have. It is incumbent upon us, as much as possible, to give the patient that knowledge, and then to accept his or her decision. It is often difficult, in cases of implied, possible, or mild cognitive impairment, to sort out whether the patient is, in fact, mentally incompetent (Fitten et al., 1984) or is simply making a decision that is not consistent with the value system of the health professionals. Some investigators have noted with psychiatric patients that the question of mental competence almost never arises, except in the case when the patient's decision conflicts with that of the physician. Decision-theory analysts have demonstrated that patients may have very different value systems from physicians. A 72-year-old woman who refused amputation for a gangrenous leg was thought to be incompetent by the surgeons, who felt she would surely die without the operation and therefore should "rationally" agree to accept the risk of surgery. A court found that she was competent and that her decision was consistent with her value system, as reflected by her entire life. She would rather have died than have had the amputation and the likely subsequent dependency. In many states, such a decision cannot even be brought to court for a competency test, except under laws applying only to the elderly. That is, if this woman had been 42 or even 59 years old, barring obviously distorted perceptions of reality and a history of mental illness, there would have been no basis on which to question her refusal; in fact, any decision to proceed would have constituted battery. One must listen to what the patient is saying and distinguish what it means to him from what it means to you. A disagreement with a proposed treatment plan does not in itself imply mental incompetence.

A third aspect of respect for persons is constituted by respectful action. When a patient is not sufficiently aware to engage in meaningful dialogue about the nature and prognosis of his or her disease, one must take care to treat that patient respectfully. This includes a range of concerns having to do with how the patient is addressed, handled, clothed, and treated during the course of hospitalization. Our actions toward those who are most vulnerable not only reflect our attitudes toward ourselves as members of the human community; they also may strengthen or instill those attitudes in others.

One also shows respect for persons in one's ambulatory practice by doing what is possible to insure that patients do not have a long wait in an uncomfortable situation, that they have ample time with the health care provider, that there is acoustical as well as visual privacy for the interaction, and, finally, that whenever possible, the patient and the physician can openly discuss the patient's concerns and wishes about his or her death and the aggressiveness of therapy in the event of severe incapacity.

Beneficence

The second principle is beneficence, which simply means doing good. It has a corollary that is an often quoted Hippocratic statement: "do no harm." The two aspects of this principle often come into conflict. The most obvious example is when a very risky or painful therapy has a chance of benefitting a patient: one wants to do good, but wonders if the more conservative route of doing no harm is not, in fact, the most ethical. It is clear that one is never required to provide treatment known to be futile: the problem is in determining how great a failure rate for a given treatment in a particular situation constitutes futility. In this particular conflict, it is, of course, whenever possible, the patient's own decision to make. In the case of an uncommunicative, comatose, or severely demented person, one is helped enormously by prior knowledge of the patient, his or her life's values, and trajectory and contributing information from family and friends.

It is important, in understanding the principle of beneficence, to distinguish doing what is best for the patient from paternalistic action. Paternalism is a stance in which one makes decisions on behalf of others, as a parent would for a child, when those persons can not decide for themselves or it is felt that they would make the wrong decisions. The history of medicine is largely one of paternalistic attitudes toward patients. It is only recently that health professionals have begun serious attempts to share medical information with their patients. The image of the caring family physician, assuming all the patient's troubles and making all the hard decisions, simply telling the patient not to worry or that "I did everything I could," is fading from view. We should not, however, reject all of the qualities of that image, for a great deal of caring concern emerges from it. In the new model of collaborative decision making, it is possible to lose the caring and beneficent aspect of health care practice to a colder and more impersonal negotiated contract. This risk is increased by physicians' fear of litigation. Previously well persons who customarily make their own decisions often adopt a passive, dependent stance when ill: illness itself may impair psychological strengths that allow for decision making. Persons who are chronically ill and have a lifetime of dependence on others' decisions may be even less able to express a preference. In such cases, when full information has been disclosed and the patient asks the physician's guidance, it is permissible to express a recommendation (Wanzer et al., 1984).

In the name of beneficence, we sometimes make decisions about letting a patient die in order to put an end to needless suffering that cannot be relieved. Merciful and compassionate treatment of the dying is a very important part of any medical practice. There are skills and knowledge in this area, including the courage and sensitivity to make the ethical decisions involved, that ought to be part of the training of every health care professional.

Justice

The third major principle is justice. Simply stated, the benefits (material and otherwise) of human society should be distributed as fairly as possible. Philosophers have found this subject a fascinating one, as it seems to be an ideal that is quite appealing to most people but not one that is easy to describe in terms of how it might actually be arrived at or carried out. Its most direct application to health care involves deliberations about allocation of scarce resources.

There is currently a great deal of discussion about the high cost of medical care and about the physician's role in keeping unnecessary costs down. This is a complex issue and a critically important one for our society, but not one that should be incorporated directly into a caring physician's decision about his or her individual patient. Obviously, one should not needlessly waste scarce resources in medicine, as in any other sphere. Nor should one expend expensive technology on a patient who has asked to be allowed to die or whom medical care cannot help. But except for these two situations, a physician who is making a decision for any patient on the basis of how much the treatment will cost is not acting strictly in the medical role. The relatonship between the physician and the patient is a fiduciary one, implying trust that the physician is acting first and foremost as the advocate of the patient. If the cost of care is the determining factor in a medical decision, what one is really saying is that the value of this patient to society does not warrant the expenditure of medical resources. This is a social perspective, and one in which our institutions should carefully weigh the fairness of distributive policies. The doctor, however, has not been trained as an arbiter of justice, nor is he or she the appropriate person to take that role. Except in war, overwhelming disasters, and other instances of dire scarcity, the rationing of health care resources must occur at the level of social policy. Health professionals should participate in the formation of that policy, but as individuals, the primary relationship should be that of loyalty toward each patient.

An example will illustrate the case of the principles of respect for persons, beneficence, and justice in ethical analysis.

An elderly demented woman who lives alone at home develops pneumonia. She is weak, cyanotic, and dyspneic; she clearly could benefit from acute hospital care, but her family refuses admission. The emergency-room staff argue that her presence there constitutes a request for treatment that calls for coercion. The family responds that they came seeking relief of her discomfort, not intravenous lines and ventilators. Resolution: an impartial third party is asked to discuss the situation with the family and patient to be sure they understand the likely consequences of each alternative and to explore other possible motives. The family is found to be able to comprehend the situation, to be realistic in their expectations, to show great devotion to the patient, and to remain adamant in their refusal of admission. They remember specific discussions she had with them before her dementia, commenting on others who died of pneumonia and on her wish to die at home. The principle of autonomy forbids coercion. The principle of respect for persons also requires that other forms of care be offered. The patient goes home with arrangements for home nursing with antibiotics and oxygen and a schedule of hospice visitors who will keep her company and see to her requests.

PRACTICAL APPROACHES TO THE ETHICAL DILEMMAS: STRATEGIES, STRUCTURES, AND SUPPORTS

The range of ethical issues raised by Alzheimer's disease is impressive and can easily be overwhelming. Ethical dilemmas are often recognized by the visceral discomfort they cause—a knotting in the stomach—or a sense of moral unease. This unease is a signal that attention needs to be paid. But it is not enough to take notice of our discomfort. Unease must lead to analysis, one which sets priorities based on ethical principles. Only through systematic analysis can an ethical basis be established for decision making and action. In ethics as in biomedicine, it is essential to be able to articulate reasons for difficult choices, especially when they are made in a context of substantial uncertainty. Nor can ethical dilemmas be resolved without reference to social policy and social ethics. To deal effectively with ethical questions requires strategies for problem solving, structures for decision making, and social supports that allow decisions to be carried out in a humane and efficient manner.

Ethics, like medicine, is both an art and a science. It is that part of philosophy which deals with systematic approaches to these kinds of problems. The approach of an ethicist includes knowledge of the philosophical principles involved as well as of their origins in cultural traditions, analysis of risk, and decision process. Much of this skill is within the reach of all health professionals and should be a part of their basic competence. There will be ethical dilemmas that are so difficult or complex that one must turn to an expert—either to an ethicist or ethics committee or to the courts. The level of basic competence includes knowing when to ask for consultation. The next section of this chapter will illustrate key steps in the ethical analysis of a clinical situation. The six key steps in the analysis are outlined first, followed by a discussion of the principles that inform our decisions.

As with other medical problems, the first step is to gather the relevant data. Information should be sought from all those involved: first and foremost the patient, and then, in the case of a patient lacking capacity to make his or her own decisions, from family, friends, nursing staff, social workers, and other involved parties. The history thus taken should be comprehensive enough to address these questions and proceed with these six steps:

1. *Factual data and conceptual clarity*—Is there a way to avoid the dilemma? Who is involved? What information is available and relevant? What missing information would make a significant difference if it were known? Is it possible to know it? For example, is information about the patient's previously expressed wishes available? Lacking that, is there guidance from the patient's lifestyle or religious affiliation?

2. *Examination of motives*—Are the motives clear? What conscious or unconscious motives may be at work—in the patient, the family, the involved health professionals? Are there family members who receive an income only as long as this patient lives? Are there health professionals involved who, being young and healthy, cannot imagine a worthwhile life at the age of 75?

3. *Application of rules or principles*—How are they selected? Can they be prioritized? What are their assumptions? Are they controversial or broadly applicable? For example, if a patient has expressed a clear preference for a certain choice in the past, that generally takes priority over quality-of-life issues.

4. *Examination of all possible consequences*—How will it affect the patient, the family, the decision makers? Any others? Are there generalizable consequences to society?

5. *Setting priorities*—Analyzing the consequences will often help clarify the basis for setting priorities among conflicting principles. This does not mean, however, that the consequences should always determine the decision—there are times when the principles will hold almost regardless of consequences. For example, the principle of preserving life in our opinion precludes administration of lethal drugs, even if the concerned parties feel "everyone would be better off that way."

6. *Making the decision*—Not to act is also to take a stance. Once one decides what to do, one must consider the best and most humane way to carry out that decision.

THE HEALTH PROFESSIONAL AS ETHICIST

Health professionals, particularly those dealing with crippling and chronic diseases such as Alzheimer's, face a barrage of ethical dilemmas in their daily work, that is, situations in which two or more conflicting ethical principles pertain to a clinical decision (Purtilo & Cassel, 1981; Veatch, 1981). For example, a confused person should be treated with respect, and yet it seems that physical restraints are needed to prevent her from falling and harming herself. It is not clear which takes priority: respect or protection. It may seem that both are important, and yet it seems we must choose one value over the other. Health practitioners frequently must decide on the spot which action is most right or least wrong. Often health care choices involve matters of life and death as well as matters of social philosophy. Given the complexities and pressures under which ethical decisions must be made, it is essential that health practitioners feel secure in their justification for making them, that they understand their own choices as outgrowths of rational, systematic analysis rather than as impulsive and inconsistent reactions.

Because many people are now surviving with profound dysfunction, disability, and dependency, there is an urgent need to focus our health care system on chronic illness and functional improvement rather than on cure (Somers, 1982). Greater longevity is a mark of success for medical science, but at the same time it creates a plethora of unique and disturbing ethical questions.

ETHICAL DILEMMAS IN ALZHEIMER'S DISEASE

Alzheimer's disease is a chronic disorder that can progress slowly or rapidly. But progress it does, over a period of years, ending eventually with death. During its course, Alzheimer patients experience debilitating health problems directly related to the disease, as well as other health problems that occur concurrently.

Ethical issues raised by Alzheimer's disease, as well as by other chronic diseases, assume a greater significance and rightfully attract greater public attention as more people survive to the age of risk for these diseases.

Cognitive impairment is the hallmark of Alzheimer's disease. This characteristic leads to a particular kind of long-term dependency and is the major source of special ethical problems. It is not enough to provide acute services for Alzheimer patients. It is essential to structure supports that will maintain function and prevent unnecessary disability. Provision of a total spectrum of long-term care in the community, acute care, and institutional care over the course of the disease is itself an ethical need. Within the process of providing such care, constant ethical decisions must be made about types of treatment—with, for, and on behalf of patients whose intelligence and personalities are disintegrating.

A major principle of medical ethics—respect for each individual's personal, free, and informed decision ("informed consent") in matters of medical care (Faden & Beauchamp, 1986)—is challenged by the difficulty of dealing with Alzheimer patients. Persons with impaired cognitive function cannot (or seem not to) understand the necessary information and may be unable to communicate a choice.

The progressive incapacity of Alzheimer patients to make decisions about their own health care collides with the strongly held presumption in our society that each individual has the right to decide what is to be done with his or her own body. The requirement of informed consent for medical treatment is the legal expression of this cultural consensus. If we were to accept the paternalistic presumption, still held in some cultures, that the physician is empowered to act on behalf of the patient rather than in concert with the patient, there would be fewer ethical dilemmas in dealing with cognitively impaired persons.

In dealing with Alzheimer's disease, health professionals are faced with an entanglement of overlapping ethical quandaries: conflict between the person's right to decide and the person's partial or total inability to decide; conflict between the responsible professional's need to provide suitable treatment and the belief that no person has the right to determine basic life (and death) choices for another; conflict between the patient's needs and interests, the needs of the family, and the scarcity of social and medical resources. These conflicts are not subtle or elusive. They require explicit analysis, ideally by a health professional who knows the patient involved, who understands basic ethical inquiry (Jonsen, 1982), and who has access to consultation from experts in law and ethics if it is necessary.

Ethical issues involved in Alzheimer's disease are aggravated by characteristics of Alzheimer patients not directly caused by the disease itself. First, Alzheimer patients belong to an already disvalued population, namely the elderly. Public awareness of the graying of America has increased, and there is growing recognition that Alzheimer's is a disease rather than a manifestation of the normal aging process. Nevertheless, attitudes toward old people have not fundamentally changed. Aging is still associated with mistaken stereotypes of disability, poverty, loneliness, and senility, even by the elderly themselves. As with other disvalued populations, such as the poor and minorities, an ethical issue of compensatory justice arises with the elderly. If we recognize this group as more vulnerable than the general population, then we must decide whether fairness demands that it be allotted a disproportionate share of resources in order to help it approach equity. Both Judeo-Christian principles of compassion and mercy and the social principle of affirmative action argue for the ethics of compensatory entitlement. But negative attitudes toward disvalued groups create resistance to allocation of resources to them. The health professional and advocate must be clear where he or she stands on this issue of ethical public policy.

Second, the growing number of Alzheimer patients must be taken into account. More than a million people in the United States now suffer from Alzheimer's disease. Because people are living longer, prevalence as well as incidence of the disease will greatly increase (see also Olsen et al., Chapter 10). This means an enormous number of people for whom substantial support systems will need to be in place. More and more families will be unable to sustain the care of these Alzheimer victims. Public responsibility on a much greater scale than now will have to be brought to bear.

The vast number of patients afflicted with Alzheimer's disease and the enormous cost of treatment act as constraints on families and professionals trying to make ethical treatment decisions on behalf of Alzheimer patients. The social core of the ethical question is this: who is to bear responsibility for the care of Alzheimer patients, and how much and what kind of care are they to get? Are we to adhere to a philosophy of rugged individualism that insists that responsibility rests with families? Or are we to consider society as a community that can and should provide resources so that severely impaired elderly persons are cared for adequately and so that their dependency does not destroy the lives of those close to them? (See also Butler, Epilogue.)

Because of the sheer number of its victims, Alzheimer's disease looms as a major arena for issues of social as well as medical ethics. Since the resources needed to care for dependent persons are social as well as medical, the resolution of the broad problem of justice here must include a notion of intergenerational responsibility, a distributive scheme that allows families to care for their own as long as is mercifully possible, and the availability of social resources for support and respite. Health care policy must be based on care for chronic as well as acute illness.

Precedents exist for dealing with populations of people lacking capacity to make their own decisions: young children, mentally retarded persons, the psychiatrically ill. Substantial efforts have been made to establish guidelines for these populations, some of which may prove applicable to Alzheimer patients (President's Commission, 1982). There are, however, limits to the similarities among these situations. Perhaps the primary distinction between intervention in cases concerning children and those involving Alzheimer patients is that the older person has a lifetime full of evidence about established value preferences.

What, then, are the ethical options for the clinician faced with medical choices when consent cannot be obtained, due to mental impairment of the patient? Some form of "proxy" consent is the first option in most cases. Two primary approaches to proxy decision making are the "best-interests" approach and the "substituted-judgment" approach. Simply put, the best-interests standard asks the health care provider in authority to decide on behalf of the patient, taking into account what is known about the values of the person who is ill. Substituted judgment is an attempt to make decisions more strictly according to the wishes of the patient. In the latter, information such as living wills, reports of expressed wishes as relayed by family and friends, and other value-relevant information, such as the spiritual or philosophical background of the person, are all taken into account. Prior arrangements such as durable power of attorney for health or a living will* are helpful in spite of their legal limitations. Without these documents the practitioner must choose between seeking *pro forma* consent to whatever he or she deems most suitable for the patient, or undergoing a painstaking and possibly futile attempt to ascertain what kind of proxy consent best represents the patient's personal values (Suber & Tabor, 1982) (see also Tune et al., Chapter 7).

With Alzheimer's disease there is a progressive but often uneven slope of decline. Borderline or fluctuating mental capacity creates difficult tensions between respect for the person's wishes and responsibility to care for a vulnerable and dependent person. The greatest pitfall in working with partially impaired persons is the temptation to judge a

---

*Editors' note: Living wills, while greatly aiding caregivers in their attempt to discover the patient's wishes, do not generally have the force of law and cannot respond flexibly to situations unanticipated at the time of their drafting. A living will is a statement of a person's future wishes for health care decisions, but it is not legally binding. A durable power of attorney for health is a written document that meets certain legal requirements and authorizes an attorney in fact, for example, a family member or friend, to make health care decisions on behalf of the principal (patient) in the event of the principal's incapacity. By designating a person to provide or withhold medical consent, the durable power of attorney allows for "substituted judgment" over a broad range of issues.

patient's choice as "incompetent" because it is based on values different from those of the decision makers.

The decisions that confront Alzheimer patients and their health practitioners include the entire range of medical and social questions, for example, whether to have elective surgery for prostatic hypertrophy, whether to take sedative medication at night to help with sleep, whether to live in sheltered housing, and whether to accept or refuse life-sustaining treatments.

The life-and-death decisions sometimes involve elaborate, sophisticated medical technology, while at other times they may center on a treatment as simple as feeding. Making these decisions on a best-interests standard raises numerous ethical questions:

1. Can one person know what is best for another?
2. Is it ethical for one person to judge what is best for another without that person's consent—possibly even in opposition to known or suspected values?
3. Often the patient and family have conflicting needs. What is the professional's responsibility in this situation? Is the family a patient as well as the diseased person?

In trying to decide life-and-death issues for seriously impaired patients, the practitioner's values about quality of life are likely to come into play. The specter of a human being losing intelligence, personality, and the ability to function as an independent person is deeply disturbing. It causes us to wonder whether a "natural" death would be preferrable to a prolongation of life that seems to us meaningless and uncomfortable. But especially in situations where the continuation of life itself is at issue, the question arises as to whether one person, even a skilled professional, can judge the quality of someone else's life and the value of its continuation. For this reason, legal and ethical standards look to substituted judgment as the best standard, especially for decisions about life-sustaining treatment (Lynn, 1984). And yet more subjective kinds of judgment can scarcely be avoided when the deterioration of the patient's condition is extreme and the cost of treatment to family and society is large in economic and emotional terms (Scitovsky & Capron, 1986).

Even if we accept the notion that health professionals faced with these dilemmas cannot avoid making judgments about quality of life, we are still caught in an ethical quagmire. What determines quality of life? Is it a certain level of human interaction? Or is it simply the absence of pain? Is lack of apparent content adequate reason to deny life-sustaining therapy? We know that with good care it is possible to keep Alzheimer patients comfortable and pain-free (Rango, 1985). But it is difficult for most people to imagine value in a vacant physiological existence cut off from meaningful recognition of self or others.

Nevertheless, the traditional stance of both medical ethics and law has been that life itself, without regard to its quality, must be sustained. Only substantial evidence of the patient's wishes could possibly justify withholding of medical measures to prolong life.

Given the fundamental importance of the principle of self-determination, advance directive strategies such as the living will and durable power of attorney become essential elements in planning ethical treatment of Alzheimer patients. By establishing the patient's choice while the patient is still able to choose, caregivers can help to see those choices respected. Although many institutions are concerned that public instances of allowing death (e.g., withholding resuscitation or termination of tube feeding) will increase their susceptibility to legal liability, this has not been the case. Most suits are brought by family members to require the physician or facility to accede to the patient's wishes to terminate treatment. Recent court decisions have upheld the importance of respect for patient autonomy whether by direct patient statement at the time of treatment or by prior directive. The Supreme Court of New Jersey, in permitting withdrawal of nasogastric tube feeding from an 84-year-old woman with multiple physical ailments and dementia, described an acceptable standard for prior directive and, where that is lacking, for a substituted judgment based on "objective" criteria. This decision also recognized quality-of-life issues, finding that excessive burden (continued and unavoidable pain) justifies the withholding of life-sustaining medical care and even nutrition. This criterion recognizes that in some cases the presumed burden of treatment as experienced by the patient outweighs its benefits (*In re* Conroy, 1985; Merritt, 1987). It is prudent that such decisions should never be easy to make and that protections against abuse exist. For this reason total legal immunity is not a reasonable goal. However, the law does provide tools for establishing and communicating the patient's values (see above, including Editor's note) and wishes that can diminish the chances of litigation.

The form of ethical philosophy that regards the doctor's relationship toward each patient as paramount would hold that in making treatment choices only the burdens to the patient should be considered. And yet, with Alzheimer's disease, the burdens to family and society appear increasingly to be considered. A false dichotomy is sometimes created between the needs of the elderly and those of other segments of society, for example, pregnant mothers or school-aged children. An ethical approach requires a recognition of our interdependence and respect for the needs of all.

Because quality of life becomes so impaired in Alzheimer patients, and because the costs of treatment for critical illness are so high, questions of life and death tend to predominate in ethical discussions. Often questions of everyday care, which deserve consideration as serious as those of life and death, are obliterated. What degree of personal care are we required ethically to perform for Alzheimer patients at each stage of their disease? Who is responsible for providing this care? Who can make decisions about the housing, feeding, and treating of Alzheimer sufferers? Such questions present themselves long before the question of sustaining or not sustaining life even arises. In the current environment of constraints in health care resources, these patients cause concern in two ways: 1) the chronic need for labor-intensive custodial care, which may go on for many years (see also Burnside, Chapter 2; Brody, Chapter 6; Reveley, Chapter 8) and 2) the use of expensive life-sustaining technologies and acute hospitalization in the event of critical illness. While decision making in critical illness has been examined extensively in recent years, the ethical issues in chronic illness and long-term care have rarely been discussed by ethicists.

One common and complex ethical issue is the question of whether to institutionalize a cognitively impaired person (Meyers DW, 1985). This issue has not received much attention in the literature of biomedical ethics. Health care professionals frequently find themselves seeking to balance their respect for a patient's free will with their concern for his or her well-being, which may require reliance upon assistance from others. In philosophical terms the health professional faces a conflict between two conflicting ethical principles: autonomy and beneficence (see above section on "Practical Approaches"). Several social mores complicate the conflict between free choice and paternalism in the context of nursing home placement.

Most people in our culture, particularly older people, have a deep aversion to nursing homes. The practicing physician may encounter an exhausted older woman who insists on caring for her dependent husband in spite of the fact that he needs round-the-clock, expert nursing care. The woman says, "I promised him I'd never put him in a nursing home." Families often feel that they are abandoning their loved ones by opting for nursing home care; and this guilt can sometimes prevent them from acting in the patient's and family's best interests. Doctors, nurses, and social workers may avoid sending patients to nursing homes out of a similar aversion, often rooted in fear of their own aging and possible dependency. In addition, they may feel a sense of professional failure when patients' needs are so extreme that they can no longer provide adequate services (Cassel & Jameton, 1981).

The decision to seek institutional long-term care can be seen from the point of view of both the patient and the family (Purtilo & Cassel, 1981). Families commonly provide extensive care to dependent elderly relatives. In the face of inadequate community support services and progressive chronic debility, the decision to seek nursing home placement is not usually reached until families have reached the limits of their endurance (see also Brody, Chapter 6).

If a more supervised living situation is required, attention should first be directed to the least restrictive alternative. Services such as respite care, adult daycare, and home health aides may permit the patient to remain at home. If it is impossible to provide support at home, the decision to pursue nursing home placement should be shared in whatever way possible with the patient. The patient should be brought along on tours of prospective homes and encouraged to express preferences. Consideration of the patient's lifelong activities and personality are directly relevant in choosing a new home.

Health care professionals who work with severely dependent patients may come to feel that the pain and suffering of the family often exceeds that of the patient. As the family turns to the physician for solace and guidance, he or she may begin to feel that the family is also a patient in need of relief from pain. Indeed, in some cases, other family members *are* regular patients of the physician, appearing at the office with back strain, depression, congestive heart failure, or other illnesses directly linked to the caregiver's role. There are several risks here. First, while grappling with the needs of the family, the physician may lose sight of the needs of the Alzheimer patient. In most cases, of course, relatives are the individuals closest and most committed to the well-being of the patient, but this should not be assumed. Family needs and desires may be at odds with the best interests of the Alzheimer patient. A family unable to give proper care may receive disability or caregiver income that will stop if the patient goes to a nursing home; an unloving relative may be eager to inherit property; an attentive spouse may be so settled in a 40-year caregiving role that fear of role change may keep aggressive treatment going long beyond the patient's wishes. A recent study of proxy consent noted that family members at times went against known wishes of the patient, which highlights some of the shortcomings of proxy (Warren et al., 1986).

Second, treating the family as a patient may intensify feelings among family members that they are needy, dependent, and incompetent to meet the demands of the situation. This is of no benefit to patient or family and may unnecessarily hasten consideration of nursing home placement. The opposite risk must also be avoided: while families are providers of care, they are not health professionals and must not be burdened with the responsibilities of trained caregivers. Explicit discussion of the physician–family relationship can clarify the obligations and limitations of all parties.

FUTURE CONCERNS

Medical institutions need to facilitate the process of ethical decision making by providing education about basic principles of bioethics, legal precedents, and current legal and political issues, and by forming ethics committees in which open discussion can take place about difficult choices. In nursing homes, proceedings concerning guardianship and other care issues must be greatly improved, with discussion of ethical issues playing a greater role.

But the largest need in dealing ethically with Alzheimer patients and their families is for social supports. Around the issue of supports, the basic social and political questions of allocation of resources and responsibility of community and society must be answered. Even with appropriate institutional structures in place, resource constraints and perverse financial incentives (such as those which favor technical intervention over personal attention) may prevent ethically correct courses from being carried out. Only with adequate social and economic supports for the care of patients with Alzheimer's disease can truly ethical treatment decisions be made.

The graying of America is, after all, a measure of the success of advanced civilization. The corollary of such success is that decisions on ethical questions in the treatment of that small percentage who are disabled and dependent ought to be made on the basis of respect for the afflicted individual's needs and value preferences and avoidance of undue personal burdens to patients and their caregivers. These two criteria must be the basis of compassionate and effective medical care and of ethical treatment decisions.

Grant support from Henry J. Kaiser Family Foundation, to Dr. Cassel.

5
One Psychiatrist's View

Gene D. Cohen

From a psychiatric viewpoint Alzheimer's disease is of great interest because, although it is a brain disorder, most of its major clinical symptoms are behavioral in nature. These behavioral symptoms fall into four general groupings: (1) cognitive dysfunction, (2) problem behaviors, (3) psychological symptoms, and (4) psychosocial stress. Cognitive dysfunctions in Alzheimer's disease are impairment of memory and intellect. Problem behaviors include wandering and agitation, the former often raising the question of nursing home placement. Psychological symptoms include depression and delusions, which define subtypes of the disorder as listed in *DSM-III-R* (American Psychiatric Association, 1987) and *ICD-9-CM* (*The International Classification of Diseases,* ninth edition, Clinical Modification, 1980). Psychosocial difficulties are reflected in the great stress experienced by families, with clinical depression disturbingly common in the caretaking relatives of Alzheimer patients.

RELATIONSHIPS BETWEEN BRAIN AND BEHAVIOR

It is indeed extraordinary that diffuse neuroanatomical and neurochemical changes occur within the brains of Alzheimer victims, while the external manifestations are so predominantly behavioral. This is what sets Alzheimer's disease apart from so many other brain disorders. With a stroke, or multiinfarct dementia, for example, the pathological changes within the brain result in identifiable physical manifestations on clinical

Drugs are listed by both brand name and generic name in the Drug Index.

examination. Signs and symptoms of nerve, motor, and muscular impairment can be elicited with strokes; electroencephalography (EEG) and computed tomography (CT scan) findings can also point to this diagnosis. But Alzheimer's disease reveals no unique or specifically diagnostic physical or laboratory findings, except on autopsy studies of brain tissue. Because of the behavioral as opposed to somatic nature of the clinical picture of Alzheimer's disease, early diagnosis presents great difficulty. Many other clinical disorders—from depression to drug side effects—can produce very similar behavioral manifestations, thereby resulting in the diagnostic confusion (Miller & Cohen, 1981). At the same time, it is this enormously underappreciated behavioral phenomenology of Alzheimer's disease that defines state-of-the-art treatment opportunities that are available today. This behavioral phenomenology defines the considerable contribution that psychiatric intervention can make in the alleviation of certain symptoms in the patient and stress in the family.

EXCESS DISABILITY AND THE IMPACT OF TREATMENT

The concept of treatment for Alzheimer's disease has been greatly misunderstood. Too often one hears that, "there is no treatment for Alzheimer's disease." What this means, however, is that there is no treatment that can cure, reverse, or stop the progression of the disorder. It does not mean that there are no treatment approaches to reduce the magnitude of the various symptoms and discomfort that accompanies the disorder. Indeed, such approaches are currently being identified (Cohen, 1983). Consider the relationship of depression to Alzheimer's disease. The question of depression begins with diagnosis. Depression alone can masquerade as Alzheimer's disease. Depression at any age can interfere with concentration and memory; in the elderly this can be especially severe. An atypical form of depression, referred to as "pseudodementia," where the magnitude and manifestations of the mood disorder are such that the patient appears to be demented, has been described in certain older adults. It has been reported that as many as 10% of older adults who are depressed look clinically as if they are demented (Roth, 1976). But it is not sufficient to ask whether an older person is presenting with depression *or* Alzheimer's disease. Research on the clinical course of such disorders has taught us that it is equally important to raise the question as to whether it could be both Alzheimer's disease *and* depression (Larson et al., 1984; see also Winograd, Chapter 1).

Studies on the manifestation of depression with Alzheimer's disease suggest that depression may occur for either of two reasons—one psychological, the other biological. Psychologically, the individual in the early and middle stages of Alzheimer's disease observes his or her own decline and can develop a reactive depression. Biologically, various neurotransmitter changes associated with affective disturbances have been identified in the brains of those who had Alzheimer's disease. While a reduction in the level of acetylcholine (ACh, a neurotransmitter associated with memory function) has been documented, a reduction in the level of norepinephrine (a neurotransmitter associated with mood states) has also been described. Hence, it appears that depression can be an actual component of the disorder, and as a result it is listed in this manner in various national and international manuals that classify diseases.

Turning this discussion around, it is important to recognize that clinicians and clinical researchers, who have for some time noted the concomitance of depression with the dementia of Alzheimer's disease, have postulated that neurotransmitters other than acetylcholine are involved in the disease process (Perry & Perry, 1985). In other words, observations of external behavioral changes, such as depression, have led some investigators to hypothesize neurochemical correlates within the brains of Alzheimer victims; such hypotheses are now appearing to be borne out. Thus, by examining the problem behaviors of these patients, we are gaining new clues about their brain pathology.

While Alzheimer's disease uncomplicated by depression causes serious memory trouble, the intellectual dysfunction is all the greater when depression accompanies the disorder. This aggravated impairment brought about by the concomitance of depression results in what investigators have labeled "excess disability"—where the patient with Alzheimer's disease does worse clinically than would ordinarily be the case (Kahn & Tobin, 1981). This excess disability has several deleterious effects. It increases the difficulty and discomfort experienced by the patient; with this greater level of dysfunction, burden on the family is increased; the diminished functional capacity of the patient then also increases the likelihood that he or she will no longer be able to reside in the community, thus increasing the risk of nursing home placement. If this excess disability can be alleviated, then the patient's discomfort decreases, family burden is reduced, and capacity to remain at home increases. Studies have shown that excess disability definitely can be modified in many patients. While the fundamental disease process in Alzheimer's disease remains difficult to modify, the ability to lift the excess disability seen with the disorder represents a treatment breakthrough. The disorder continues in a progressive manner, but the impact on all involved can be lessened.

LESSONS FROM HISTORY: ALOIS ALZHEIMER'S CLASSIC CASE

Many of the same clinical consequences of depression causing excess disability can be seen in the delusions that can accompany Alzheimer's disease. The classic case of the disorder described by Alois Alzheimer in 1907 was a woman who was brought in for help by her husband because of her paranoid delusions and other disturbing behavioral symptoms (Alzheimer, 1907). In 1906, at a meeting of the Association of Southwest German Specialists in Mental Diseases, Alzheimer presented a report, from which the following excerpt has been taken and translated. The cognitive, behavioral, psychological, and psychosocial aspects of Alzheimer's disease are all illustrated in this brief excerpt:

> A woman 51 years of age exhibited ideas of jealousy against her husband as the first notable symptom. Soon a rapidly progressing loss of memory became apparent; she could no longer find her way around her home, dragged objects back and forth, hid them; at times she believed someone wanted to kill her and began to shout loudly.

The occurrence of psychotic or paranoid symptoms in conjunction with the dementia of Alzheimer's disease often brings about a situation of triple jeopardy for the family. First, the family is already experiencing anguish over the cognitive deterioration of their loved one; second, the family suffers physical and economic burdens in providing care; third, if delusions occur—especially those leading to paranoid thoughts about the caregiver—then the family not only fails to receive expressions of appreciation from the patient, but might receive accusations instead. This can be the straw that breaks the family's capacity to care for a loved one in the community. The absence of appreciation combined with paranoid accusations perhaps explains the high prevalence of depression in spouses of Alzheimer victims (Zarit et al., 1985). What one is witnessing here is another situation of excess disability—excess disability on the part of patient and family alike. Psychiatric interventions can alleviate this excess disability as well. Such approaches may include behavioral techniques, psychotherapy (particularly in the early to middle stages of the disorder), and, at times, the judicious use of psychotropic medications (Reisberg, 1983).

APPROACHES TO TREATMENT

Two brief, relatively mild examples illustrate the nature of the problem and the opportunity to treat excess disability in Alzheimer's disease. While these examples focus on patients in the early and middle stages of Alzheimer's disease, it should be kept in mind that treatment approaches that alter symptomatology and suffering can be employed throughout the entire course of the disorder (Cohen, 1983).

CASE 1: A 75-year-old brilliant chemist, Professor JB, was evaluated because of significant trouble he was having with memory and concentration—to the extent that he no longer could balance his checkbook and no longer took an interest in reading. Professor JB described a difficulty noticeable only to him, a year earlier, when he found himself becoming less facile with complicated equations. To others he still looked quite sharp, but not to himself. This problem was a terrible blow to Professor JB's self-esteem, and he began to experience trouble sleeping, loss of appetite and weight, and further difficulty concentrating. A thorough differential diagnostic workup ruled out many causes of dementia-like symptoms that can mimic senile dementia, leaving the clinician with the diagnosis of Alzheimer's disease. But the impression was that depression was also present.

Treatment was instituted for the depression, combining individual psychotherapy and an antidepressant medication. Professor JB's appetite returned, the weight loss stopped, concentration improved, and he started reading again; his difficulties with his checkbook, however, continued. The therapeutic work helped him come to terms with his underlying disorder, with Alzheimer's disease. Residual skills were maximized during that stage of his illness; quality of life during that interval was enhanced.

Dramatically illustrated in this example is the remarkable phenomenon of a patient experiencing temporary restoration of function while suffering from an underlying progressive illness—the impact of lifting excess disability. Following the intervention for depression, another three years passed before the level of cognitive impairment with which Professor JB was first seen returned. Treatment gave him three better years at a critical juncture in his life course.

CASE 2: Mrs. TM, a 76-year-old woman with Alzheimer's disease, who had lost her husband three years earlier, was having increasing difficulty managing her two-bedroom condominium by herself. She had a daughter who worked and an older sister living in the vicinity, providing her emotional support and help with some of her household responsibilities. However, her increasing incapacity, together with the limits in her daughter's time and her sister's strength, made it necessary for the family to seek home help for Mrs. TM. An effort was made to engage the services of a homemaker. Mrs. TM resisted this idea, saying that she valued her independence and was sure that a stranger would only interfere in her affairs. She finally relented, but the homemaker was allowed to come for only a week, at which point Mrs. TM told her not to come back. She was defensive about her actions, exclaming that the homemaker was planning to steal her belongings. Efforts to get her to accept a new homemaker proved futile, and the family wondered whether she would be able to continue living alone under the circumstances. At the same time, Mrs. TM was very resistant to the idea of moving.

Consultation was sought, and Mrs. TM consented to be examined in her apartment. In addition to a mild to moderate degree of memory impairment and difficulty in following through with various chores, Mrs. TM revealed covert paranoid thinking that became apparent only on careful probing. She had subtle but significant concerns about a conspiracy going on among unknown parties, aimed at taking over her holdings. The delusions were not challenged (which would likely only have provoked the patient at that point and caused her to lose confidence in the therapist); the inner tension that she felt about them was real (since both fantasy and reality can stir great anxiety) and was accordingly acknowledged. This acknowledgment became the basis of a therapeutic alliance that permitted her to accept the idea of trying some medication to help her better cope with the stress of her situation. A small dose of antipsychotic medication was prescribed in conjunction with follow-up supportive psychotherapeutic visits. The delusions subsided, and Mrs. TM allowed the idea of homemaker assistance to be brought up again. This time she was able to tolerate a stranger coming into her home, and the arrangement worked out. Mrs. TM died four years later, from a heart attack at home.

This case illustrates the degree to which delusions can compound coping capacity in Alzheimer's disease, showing what improvement can follow if these delusions can be lifted or lightened. Also illustrated is how, allowing for varying durations to the clinical course of Alzheimer's disease in different individuals, one might die *with* the disease (from other causes) at a less advanced stage, rather than *from* it (as many have suggested) at an advanced stage (see also Winograd, Chapter 1). In this case, too, treatment gave the patient better years—with less symptomatology and a higher level of functioning—than would otherwise have been the situation in the course of her illness.

REIMBURSEMENT CHANGE FOR ALZHEIMER'S DISEASE AND RELATED DISORDERS

A recent change in Medicare reimbursement policy extends the availability of psychiatric treatment for Alzheimer patients. In September of 1984 a major task force report on Alzheimer's disease was released by the U.S.

Department of Health and Human Services. Within the report there was a "special financing recommendation" that was announced as being implemented in conjunction with the release of the report (U.S. Department of Health and Human Services, 1984a). Some have regarded this development as "the most important change in Medicare coverage for mental disorders since the inception of Medicare" over 20 years ago (Goldman et al., 1985, p. 939). Before this, reimbursement for psychotherapy was limited to $250 per year, an amount that had not changed since the original legislation was enacted in 1965. The purpose of the recommendation was to "remove limitations on some services for Alzheimer's disease and related disorders provided outside the hospital setting." Specifically, the recommendation reads as follows:

> Current Medicare statute limits medically appropriate physician services provided outside of the hospital setting for patients with Alzheimer's disease when coded as a mental disorder. The Department should clarify that, except for psychotherapy, physician treatment services for patients with Alzheimer's disease and related disorders are not subject to the $250 limitations. In other words, in determining whether services for these patients are subject to the limit, the nature of the physician's service is the deciding factor, not the diagnostic code. Therefore, physician treatment services provided outside the hospital setting for patients with Alzheimer's disease and related disorders coded 290.X (in *DSM-III* and *ICD-9-CM*) should be reimbursed in the same manner as services for Alzheimer's disease coded 331*(ICD-9-CM)* (U.S. Dept. of Health and Human Services, 1984a, page xv).*

The intent of this administrative change was to correct an inconsistency where reimbursement for the same service differed, depending on which diagnostic code for the treatment of Alzheimer's disease was used (290.X vs. 331), although both codes referred to Alzheimer's disease and related disorders. The intent, too, was to reimburse for office visits for the medical management of Alzheimer's disease (including pharmacotherapy and other nonpsychotherapy treatment interventions) on an 80:20 reimbursement/copayment formula, as opposed to the $250 limit and 50:50 reimbursement/copayment formula that unfortunately still holds for psychotherapy. The change was also motivated by a recognition of

---

*Editors' note: The *DSM-III* and *ICD-9-CM* are internationally accepted numerical codes for categorization of diseases and medical disorders. The *DSM-III* (now *DSM-III-R*) is used for psychiatric and psychological classification. The *ICD-9-CM* is used for the indexing of hospital records by disease and operation and the classification of morbidity and mortality information for statistical purposes. The 290 classification is for organic mental syndromes of dementias arising in the senium and presenium. The X indicates that there are additional subcategories within the classification. The 331 classification in ICD-9-CM is only for cerebral degenerative diseases of the central nervous system. Both classifications include Alzheimer's disease.

the behavioral nature of much of the clinical pathology of Alzheimer's disease and the major role of psychiatric interventions in the treatment process. This change should play a useful role in improving the ability of those organic mental disorder patients with Alzheimer's disease or a related disorder to seek state-of-the-art clinical intervention, though the continuing limitation on psychotherapy reimbursement may lead to over-reliance on pharmacotherapy.

THE ROLE OF PSYCHOTHERAPY IN THE TREATMENT OF ALZHEIMER'S DISEASE

While the Medicare change discussed above allows for improved coverage of psychiatric interventions other than psychotherapy in the treatment of Alzheimer's disease, the potential role of psychotherapy for certain Alzheimer patients and their families can be a very important one. Too often the potential contribution of supportive psychotherapy to an overall treatment plan is overlooked or misunderstood with this disorder. Indeed, in both case examples above, supportive psychotherapy was alluded to and played an important part in alleviating symptoms and improving the clinical course.

The appropriateness of psychotherapeutic interventions extends to both patient and family in coping with Alzheimer's disease. Professor JB in Case 1 above typifies many Alzheimer patients, who are painfully aware of their cognitive deficits and functional impairments in the early stages of the disorder. Depressive symptomatology in response to these losses and accompanying threats to self-esteem are common and can be alleviated via supportive psychotherapeutic interventions. Psychodynamic understanding can assist in this process, particularly in dealing with troubling clinical manifestations of psychological defense mechanisms (as with Mrs. TM in Case 2 above) in these patients (Verwoerdt, 1981). The ramifications of alleviating excess disability and enhancing the quality of life for the Alzheimer patient have already been elaborated; supportive psychotherapy can contribute to this key intervention opportunity.

Psychotherapeutic and related psychodynamic issues apply to families throughout the entire course of Alzheimer's disease. The disturbingly high frequency of reactive depression among close relatives of Alzheimer victims has been increasingly documented. The elements of loss with potentially severe emotional consequences are multiple among spouses of victims. Diminished capacities for intellectual exchange, empathic sharing, and sexual fulfillment all take their toll. Intense feelings of guilt, often without basis, can be extremely stressful. Family members may inappropriately feel guilty about somehow causing their loved one's disease; they often feel guilty when they experience frustration or anger in facing their overwhelming responsibilities as caregivers; they commonly suffer guilt feelings when exploring nursing home placement, even when such an arrangement is long overdue; the burden of guilt feelings and a sense of helplessness may be unconsciously projected into anger toward nursing home staff or other health care providers, thereby generating still further stress. Psychotherapeutic consultations can offer families considerable opportunities for emotional catharsis, understanding of ambivalent feelings, and perspective on the inevitable mix of troubling thoughts and affect that can accompany care of an Alzheimer patient (see also Tune et al., Chapter 7).

SUMMARY

More than eight decades after Alzheimer's classic case, the behavioral problems that form much of the basis for treatment in Alzheimer's disease are beginning to gain some measure of attention along with the associated brain changes that cause them. Both brain and behavior changes in Alzheimer's disease must command our attention, for purposes of both research and treatment.

The opinions expressed herein are those of the author and not necessarily those of the Veterans Administration.

PART II
Family and Community Interventions

6
The Long Haul:
A Family Odyssey

Elaine M. Brody

The major burden of caring for people with Alzheimer's disease and related disorders rests and will continue to rest with their families. The most dedicated and sophisticated professional efforts cannot succeed without the backup of caregivers who, in the final analysis, are the ones confronted with the "long haul." Family members, most often the central caregivers, face the ongoing, unrelenting, time-extended daily task of maximizing the patient's functional capacities. Their role just begins when the professional assessment process has been completed, diagnoses, have been made, and treatment plans have been formulated.

Since the family is relied upon for the practical implementation of professional recommendations, assessment of the patient's capacities should be accompanied by assessment of the family's capacities to meet identified needs. To do so, attention must be focused on the experiences and problems of family members themselves, the effects on their lives of caring for their cognitively impaired relatives, and *their* needs for help and care.

In short, from the perspective of professionals, family members play two roles: they are *partners* in the caring enterprise and they are *clients/ patients* as well (see also Tune et al., Chapter 7).

FAMILIES AS PARTNERS IN CARE

Research on family caregiving to the elderly has yielded a body of information so consistent that it is no longer at issue. Certain facts are therefore accepted here as givens and will be summarized very briefly (Brody EM, 1985b; Horowitz, 1985a):

1. Families of disabled older people have an excellent record in providing care; they do indeed care for and about their elderly family members (see also Reveley, Chapter 8).

2. Families (not the formal system of government, agencies, and professionals) provide more than 80% of medically related care and home nursing, hands-on personal care, household maintenance, transportation, and shopping (Comptroller General of the United States, 1977a; Shanas, 1979a, 1979b, 1980). In addition, families respond in emergencies, provide intermittent acute care, and receive the elderly when they are discharged from hospitals and other facilities.

3. Families provide the emotional support—the concern, affection, socializing, and sense of having someone on whom to rely—that is the most universal family service and is the form of family help most wanted by the old.

4. Services from the formal support system do not encourage families to shirk caregiving. Rather, they complement and supplement family services, strengthening the family's capacity to do what it has been trying to do (Horowitz, 1982; Zimmer & Sainer, 1978). Moreover, when formal services are offered, families are extremely modest in their requests.

5. The family mobilizes, coordinates, and monitors family and formal services, a form of help that is often regarded as the province of professionals and characterized as "case management."

6. Families do not dump ill relatives into nursing homes. Most often, institutional placement is preceded by a prolonged and exhausting haul during which strenuous efforts are made to keep the disabled person in the community (Brody EM, 1969; Brody & Gummer, 1967; Townsend, 1965).

Family care of the elderly is not a new phenomenon, of course. However, the radical demographic developments in this century—in particular, the vast increase in the number and proportion of very old people who are vulnerable to Alzheimer's disease and other chronic ailments—have resulted in a very long and difficult haul indeed for many more families than used to be the case (see also Williams, Chapter 9; Olsen et al., Chapter 10; Butler, Epilogue). Since those demographic trends will continue, the number of families confronted with the long haul will inevitably rise unless a dramatic breakthrough occurs to prevent, ameliorate, or cure Alzheimer's disease.

Until now the family has met the challenge of providing care with relatively little help from professionals or social and governmental agencies. For example, recent data from the 1982 Health Care Financing Administration (HCFA) Long-Term Care Survey show that less than 15% of all "helper days of care" to people needing help with activities of daily living (ADLs), an extreme form of caregiving, are provided by the formal system. Moreover, these data show that only 4% of old people who need such help have any part of it paid for by government (Doty et al., 1985); that is, most of the help purchased is paid for by the patients and their families (Brody EM & Schoonover, 1986).

The indications are that families will continue to be reliable partners in care and will remain committed to caring. Attitudes of the younger generations, which are clues to the future, show no weakening of the value that care of the elderly is a family responsibility (Brody EM et al., 1983).

THE FAMILY AS PATIENT

Caregiving to the disabled elderly is not without social cost, however. Many recent studies of the effects of caregiving on family caregivers lead to the inescapable conclusion that such family members should be regarded by professionals as *patients* as well as *partners* in care (see also Winograd, Chapter 1; Tune et al., Chapter 7).

The impact of caregiving on family members depends on individual and family characteristics. There is enormous variability in the qualities and situations of caregivers and families. The dependent person may be a spouse, a parent, a parent-in-law, a sibling, a grandparent, an aunt, or an uncle. In general, the informal support network tends to be structured hierarchically, based primarily on the service provider's relationship to the dependent person (spouse, near kin, distant kin, and friends), but also on geographic proximity. Spouses, children, and children-in-law play central roles for most of the dependent elderly. Daughters and daughters-in-law are the most prevalent helpers to people with disabled spouses and to widowed older people (Brody EM, 1981b; Horowitz, 1982; Myllyluoma & Soldo, 1980; Shanas, 1979b). For the most part, friends and neighbors play much smaller roles in the helping network. Although they are important resources when children are absent or unavailable, their efforts usually do not approach those of family members in duration or intensity (Cantor, 1979; Johnson, 1979; Stoller & Earl, 1983). Friends and neighbors often do, however, serve to link the elderly to needed services in the community (New York State Health Advisory Council, 1981).

Beyond the degree of relatedness, many other variables are relevant to the level of caregiving provided—for example, family structure; the quality of relationship between afflicted person and caregiver; economic resources; other demands on family members' time and energy; and urban/rural, socioeconomic, and ethnic factors (see also Winograd, Chapter 1).

In the main, the distribution of the various kinds of tasks among informal providers is gender-specific and/or based on degree of relatedness. Personal care (bathing, dressing, feeding, etc.) and instrumental services (household tasks, shopping, transportation, etc.) are provided by spouses when the disabled person is married, often helped by adult daughters. When the person needing help is widowed or divorced, daughters predominate in providing concrete services and are three times more likely than sons to share their households with a dependent elderly parent (Brody EM, 1978, 1981b; Horowitz, 1982; Myllyluoma & Soldo, 1980; Shanas, 1979b; Stoller, 1983; Troll, 1971). Sons tend to play a larger role in helping with certain gender-defined services, such as money management and decision making (Stoller, 1983; Treas, 1977; Horowitz, 1985b), and become the "responsible relatives" for those who have no daughters or none close by. Both sons and daughters provide their parents with emotional support (Horowitz, 1985b).

Caregiving Spouses

Due to the difference between the sexes in life expectancy and the tendency of men to marry women younger than themselves, elderly men with Alzheimer's disease are much more likely than elderly women to have spouses on whom to rely. Most of the 9 million widowed older people are women. At age 65 and over, more than half of older women (52%) are widowed, while more older men (77%) are married.* Rates of widowhood rise sharply with advancing age, and the imbalance in the proportions of women to men increases. Between the ages of 65 and 74, the ratio of women to men is 131 : 100; between 75 and 84 the ratio is 166 : 100; and at age 85 and over there are 224 women to every 100 men (Allan & Brotman, 1981).

Whether they are husbands or wives, most older people exert extreme efforts to care for a disabled spouse, but their capacities are often limited by their own advanced age, reduced energy and strength, and age-related ailments. Compared with other relatives who provide care,

*Editors' Note: Data on the impact of divorce are lacking. As a factor affecting caregiving spouses, divorce is bound to assume increasing importance as we approach the twenty-first century.

spouses experience the most stress (Shindelman et al., 1981). Wives who care for disabled husbands, for example, have been found to suffer from low morale, isolation, loneliness, economic hardship, and "role overload" due to multiple responsibilities (Fengler & Goodrich, 1979). Such caregivers, therefore, require close attention to their own needs for respite (temporary relief from caregiving activities), concrete helping services, and emotional support. Since more couples nowadays survive together into advanced old age, such situations are likely to occur with increasing frequency.

Caregiving Adult Children

When an elderly couple has children, they assist the "well" spouse in caring for the disabled parent; when an older person is widowed, the bulk of care is given by adult children (Shanas, 1979a; Sussman, 1965; Tobin SS & Kulys, 1980). Though most older people prefer to live in their own households, about 18% of the elderly live with their children, primarily because they cannot live alone (Shanas, 1979a). These are cross-sectional data, however; that is, data taken at one point in time. Older people tend to move into their children's households because disabilities (including Alzheimer's disease) make it impossible for them to manage on their own. The result is that many more than the 18% of older people indicated by cross-sectional data share a child's home at *some* point in their lives.

Looking at shared households from the perspective of adult children, Soldo (1980) estimates (again, based on cross-sectional data) that more than 1.7 million women in their forties and fifties have an elderly person in their homes and more than an additional half million have both an elderly person and a child under 18 in their households. That figure does not include sons who share households, adult children of either sex who are either under 40 or over 60, or households with children over the age of 18. A conservative estimate, therefore, is that there are at least a million three-generation households, in many of which the elderly person has Alzheimer's disease.

Since parents and children age together, the adult children of the increasing number of people in advanced old age are most often themselves either in middle or old age. While the peak parent-care years appear to be when people are in their late forties and fifties, about one-third are either under 40 or over 60. Torrey (1985) reports that the median age of the children of an 85-year-old woman is 59. The need to provide parent care, then, occurs at a time of life when the adult children themselves may be experiencing age-related interpersonal losses, the onset of chronic ailments, lower energy levels, and retirement or approaching retirement. Their responsibilities often extend both upward to the old and downward to the younger generation.

The need to care for the old arises for many women at a time when most people expect to have "empty nests" but find that those empty nests are refilled (literally or in terms of increased responsibility) by impaired older people in need of care (Brody EM, 1978). As women advance from 40 years of age to their early sixties, for example, those who have a surviving parent are more likely to have that parent be dependent on them, to spend more time caring for the parent, to perform more difficult caregiving tasks, and to have the parent in their own household (Lang & Brody EM, 1983). Middle-aged children, then, may not only be experiencing their own age-related problems; their responsibilities may peak rather than diminish at this stage in their lives.

Younger caregivers may still have their own children at home. The steady trend to delay childbearing to later ages means that in the future more people will arrive at the parent-care years while they have young children at home. Between 1972 and 1983, for example, the first-birth rate for women in their thirties more than doubled (National Center for Health Statistics, 1985). In one recent study, two-thirds of caregiving daughters had children living at home, most under 18 years of age and some (10%) younger than six (Brody EM, 1985b). Beyond anecdotal reports (see, for example, Brody EM, in press), there has been virtually no exploration of the effects on grandchildren of having a dependent older person living in the household (whether or not the grandparent has Alzheimer's disease).

Effects of Family Caregiving

Research on the effects of family caregiving began with the classic Sainsbury and Grad de Alarcon studies in Great Britain (Sainsbury & Grad de Alarcon, 1970) and has been accelerating recently. The findings of various studies are consistent in speaking to the role of caregivers as patients.

While some caregivers report that they experience financial hardship (about 15–20%) or declines in their physical health (about 25%), study after study (Horowitz, 1985a) has identified the most pervasive and most severe consequences as being in the realm of emotional strains (see also Winograd, Chapter 1). Mental health symptoms such as depression, anxiety, frustration, helplessness, sleeplessness, lowered morale, and emotional exhaustion are related to restrictions on time and freedom, isolation, conflict from the competing demands of various responsibilities, difficulties in setting priorities, and interference with lifestyle and social and recreational activities (see Archbold, 1978; Cantor, 1983; Danis, 1978; Frankfather et al., 1981; Gurland et al., 1978; Hoenig & Hamilton, 1966; Horowitz, 1982; Robinson & Thurnher, 1979). Such findings are not unique to the United States. Similar information is emerging from other countries (Gibson MJ, 1982; Horl & Rosenmayr, 1982).

Caregiving daughters appear to be more vulnerable to such negative effects than sons. When sons become principal caregivers they do less, are helped by their wives, and experience less strain (Horowitz, 1985b). The vulnerability of daughters to caregiving strains may be due to their socialization as nurturers and the feeling that it is *their* responsibility to provide all the care needed (Brody EM, 1985b). In addition, they are more likely than sons to be subject to the multiple competing demands of home, family, parent care, and work. Such women have been characterized as "women-in-the-middle" (Brody EM, 1981b). Not only do the pressures they experience place them at high risk for mental and physical health symptoms, but their stress affects other family members as well. Among the family strains that have been identified are relationship problems, lack of privacy, changed routines, and postponement of vacations and future plans.

Very recently, attention has been called to another kind of cost to the family that is a consequence of caregiving. Some caregiving daughters leave their jobs or cut back on working hours because of the care needs of elderly husbands and parents, resulting in sharp reductions in family income (Brody EM, 1985b; Brody EM et al., 1987). Some caregiving spouses and adult children are deterred from participation in the labor force (Soldo & Myllyluoma, 1983). Recent findings from the HCFA Long-Term Care Survey (with a nationally representative sample) indicate that 11.6% of caregiving daughters, 5% of caregiving sons, 13.5% of caregiving wives, and 11.4% of caregiving husbands had left their jobs to take care of an elderly person (Stone et al., in press). Even higher proportions had cut back on working hours, taken time off without pay, or rearranged their work schedules. Similarly, a British survey found that among women between the ages of 40 and 59, the need to look after people other than their husbands was second only to ill health as a reason for giving up work. Nineteen percent of women in their forties and 14% of those in their fifties were in that category (Hunt, 1978).

Information about the effects of women's workforce participation on the care of elderly parents is beginning to emerge. Scattered findings indicate that working women continue to meet their responsibilities to their families, their elderly parents, and their jobs, but give up their own free time and opportunities for socializing (Cantor, 1983; Horowitz et al., 1983; Lang & Brody EM, 1983). One recent study found that disabled parents of working women and nonworking women received the same amount of care from all sources of services together (Brody EM & Schoonover, 1986). Employed and nonworking daughters provided equal amounts of emotional support, service arrangement and financial management, shopping and transportation. When the daughters worked, however, the family purchased more help for personal care, but there was no increase in the utilization of services subsidized by governmental agencies.

Caregiving to Alzheimer Patients

It is generally agreed that caring for an Alzheimer patient presents extraordinary difficulties that derive from many sources. The symptoms themselves are singularly distressing to the people who care for and about the person—symptoms such as confusion, forgetfulness, disorientation, incontinence, combativeness (even violence), and abrupt swings of mood. Perhaps most distressing of all is the loss of the person herself or himself as an individual with whom one can communicate, who can provide feedback to the caregiver that his or her efforts have some effect and are appreciated.

Such symptoms translate into special needs for care. The patient often cannot be left alone, frequently requiring 24-hour surveillance. The caregiver may, therefore, be isolated, and the entire family's lifestyle may be disrupted. Under these conditions caregivers often experience anxiety about their own future. They wonder: Does this run in families? Will I (or other family members) get Alzheimer's some day? How long will this go on? What future is there for the patient? for me and for other members of my family? And they feel guilty because of very human feelings they experience but may not be able to express or acknowledge even to themselves—feelings of resentment, anger, and even the wish to be rid of the heavy burdens they carry (see also Tune et al., Chapter 7).

Few research studies have focused on the effects of caregiving that are unique when the old person's diagnosis is Alzheimer's disease. Taken together, however, scattered research findings and many clinical reports indicate that caregiving to patients with that diagnosis does have special features and is a strong predictor of strain. Sharing a household with an impaired older person is another strong predictor of strain, and shared households are often the outcome of the older person's cognitive impairment.

One study that focused specifically on caregivers to memory-impaired adults found that spouses, followed closely by adult children, had the lowest levels of well-being compared with caregivers to patients with other diagnoses (George, 1983). Spouses of these patients took the most psychotropic drugs. As in other studies, shared living arrangements predicted more stress symptoms and lower levels of well-being. The greatest caregiver burden was in the areas of mental health and social participation, with about 60% of the caregivers expressing a need for more help.

The George study also compared caregivers of memory-impaired adults with age-matched peers who did not have caregiving responsibilities, finding caregivers to have three times as many symptoms of stress. They were not compared, however, with caregivers to people with other kinds of disabilities. Therefore no conclusions can be drawn as to the differential effects on caregivers of helping Alzheimer patients versus helping patients with other diagnoses.

OPTIONS FAMILIES CHOOSE

When confronted with the long haul of a cognitively impaired relative, families take diverse paths as the disease progresses and the difficulties of providing care increase. The course of Alzheimer's is believed to be an average of six to 10 years from onset till death (see also Williams, Chapter 9). That timeframe should not obscure the fact that in some cases the caregiving odyssey is even longer and, in many instances, caregiving had been going on for other reasons for long periods of time *before* Alzheimer's disease made its appearance.

When the symptoms of Alzheimer's do appear, the family begins a new phase in its prolonged period of adaptation and coping. Professional help may be sought to find out what is wrong, but unsophisticated families may assume that the symptoms are part of a process of aging that is to be expected and thus may do nothing. The caregiving process often begins by monitoring the disabled person with frequent telephone checks and visits. Gradually, the family finds it necessary to manage money and unattended checkbooks, do neglected housekeeping, attempt to remedy inadequate and irregular meals or poor personal hygiene, do the shopping, and provide transportation. The pace of caregiving may then be quickened by a dramatic event that signals the need for more intensive care and supervision and puts an end to the disabled person's independent living. The patient is picked up at night by the police, or enters neighbors' homes uninvited, or starts a fire by leaving the stove unwatched. Since few families can afford to purchase round-the-clock in-home care, Alzheimer patients without spouses then may be brought to the home of an adult child.

Studies at the Philadelphia Geriatric Center have been exploring the differential effects of caregiving on daughters who are employed and those who are not. What is important in the context of this book is that women who had left their jobs or had cut back on their working hours because of competition between work and parent care had the most severely disabled mothers and *mothers who more often had Alzheimer's disease or a related disorder* (Brody EM et al., 1984b). As might be expected, both the caregiving daughters and their mothers were older and more often shared a household than the other women studied. The health of the women who quit their jobs had suffered, they had been providing care for long periods of time, and they had the lowest family incomes. The women who had cut back their working hours showed the effects of competing demands on them. Some had lost time from work or had passed up opportunities for advancement, they had less time for themselves and their husbands, and they felt they had missed out on something.

In the same study, when the daughters reported feeling depressed as a result of caregiving, the sources of depression were different for working and nonworking women (Hoffman et al., 1984). Reports of depression by the women who had reduced the number of working hours were associated with their *mothers' symptoms of Alzheimer's disease*. These daughters also reported worrying about their ability to care for their mothers in the future. Undoubtedly their mothers' cognitive problems augured increased caregiving demands and lifestyle changes, a future in which the daughters might find themselves unable to cope with their multiple responsibilities. A predictor of depression for the nonworking women was having given up their jobs to care for their mothers.

INTERVENTION PROGRAMS

In recent years, as studies of caregivers have documented the burdens experienced, a variety of intervention programs have been developed that aim to decrease the strains. Such programs include those designed to increase the caregivers' knowledge about the older person's disability and/or to provide social support (e.g., lectures, discussion groups); concrete services such as daycare, respite, and home health services; self-help groups; and psychotherapeutic help. It is probable that families do experience benefits as a result of such programs, and both staff and families report such benefits anecdotally. However, Gallagher's excellent review (1985) of the literature on these strategies concludes that ". . . the literature . . . on the effectiveness of caregiver support and/or educational programs can, at best, be regarded as relatively sparse and primarily impressionistic" (p. 259).

Few such programs are specific to families of Alzheimer patients. The most visible of these are the self-help support groups that have proliferated across the country under the aegis of the Alzheimer's Disease and Related Disorders Association (ADRDA). Though empirical data are lacking to verify the reduction in burden that may result from participation, the popularity of the groups indicates that caregivers perceive participation in the groups to be helpful. Some professionals express concern, however, about participants whose emotional problems may be exacerbated in groups without skilled professional leadership (see also Tune et al., Chapter 7; Reveley, Chapter 8; Sainer, Chapter 11).

A respite program specifically for families caring for Alzheimer patients is currently underway at the Philadelphia Geriatric Center. The project has a randomized control group design and offers a variety of respite care, including temporary nursing home care, in-home respite, and daycare.

It is well known that helping services are underdeveloped and by no means universally available. However, there are problems that require attention even when services can be obtained. To help them in their long haul, some families avail themselves of formal services (where they exist) and some do not. Those who do not use services may lack information or money, but they often fail to do so because of psychological barriers such as guilt or the desire for total control over the situation.

The challenge, then, is not only to develop and fund services, but also to help families with problems that prevent them from using services that exist. It is simplistic to put our faith in channeling, information and referral, or case management without attending to the counseling or psychotherapeutic service that is the critical ingredient enabling families to use other services. Whatever label is given to coordinating and linking services, they must be accompanied by individualized attention to psychological, financial, and social barriers to getting help and to the intrapsychic and interpersonal problems that exist (see also Tune et al., Chapter 7).

In a climate in which the emphasis is on encouraging family members to provide care and on training them in caregiving skills (such training should be done, of course), it should also be kept in mind that all caregiving does not represent family cohesiveness or healthy behavior. When families continue to provide unrelenting, prolonged, extraordinarily difficult care to the extent that their own health and well-being and that of other family members suffer severely, their perseverance and endurance may indicate that something is very wrong. The help such families need should not take the form of encouraging caregiving but should aim to identify the nature of the problem and to help the family find more adaptive solutions, even if it means a reduction in its caregiving.

The Elderly Without Close Family

Elderly individuals without family or whose family members are not close at hand, and whose illness or disability is severe and likely to be prolonged, are at high risk. They therefore require special attention from formal system providers.

A significant minority of older people do not have a close family member on whom to rely. The proportion who are deprived in that respect rises with advancing age. At age 74 and over, for example, 68% of women and 24% of men are widowed, in addition to the 9% of women and 7% of men who are divorced or have never married. About 20% of people who are now 65 and over have never had a child, and an undetermined number are childless because they have outlived their children (Allan & Brotman, 1981). Although the vast majority of those with children see them frequently, 11% (almost 2 million old people) do not see a child as often as once a month (Shanas, 1979b). For most of these, geographic distance precludes the availability of a child for day-to-day supportive health care; for a minority, little or no help can be expected due to longstanding alienation. Overall, more than one in 20 (5.3%) of all people 65 and over are entirely kinless—that is, without spouse, children, or siblings.*

In the future there are likely to be more ailing older people without close family ties. The birthrate continues to fall. There will be fewer children among people who have children and more people who have no children (National Center for Health Statistics, 1985).

---

*Editors' Note: The data on kinship and family support were gathered in the 1970s. Changes in these patterns can be expected with the demographic shifts anticipated in the last decades of the twentieth century.

Family Relationships of the Institutionalized Aged

Despite the widespread notion that old people are dumped into nursing homes by hardhearted uncaring families, research has definitively established that such placement is made only after the families have made prolonged and strenuous efforts to avoid it. Alzheimer patients constitute a substantial percentage of those who reside in nursing homes.

The 5% of those 65 and over who are in institutions at any one time are outnumbered two to one by equally disabled noninstitutionalized old people who are cared for by their families (Brody SJ et al., 1978; Comptroller General of the United States, 1977b). Moreover, this proportion did not change between 1962 and 1975 despite important social changes that took place during that time (Shanas, 1979b). The role of social support in the form of family is highlighted by the fact that, in contrast to those who live in the community, the vast majority (88%) of the institutionalized aged are not married (being widowed, divorced, or never married), half are childless, and those who have children have fewer children than the noninstitutionalized (Brody EM, 1981b).

When families go beyond the limits of their endurance, one option should be the availability of quality nursing home care. It cannot be assumed that all Alzheimer patients are better off in the community. One study found that the bleakness and deprivation of the lives of some patients living in the community amounted to almost total desolation (Brody, 1985a). They were confined to their homes; most never left their bedrooms, even to eat. Most spent their days without any stimulation at all—doing virtually nothing but sleeping, lying in bed, and talking to themselves. Such extremely impaired people are the ones most neglected by agencies whose mission it is to deliver diversional or recreational services (Comptroller General of the United States, 1977a, 1977b).

Weissert's comprehensive and definitive analysis (Weissert, 1985) indicates that for severely impaired people such as Alzheimer patients, community care is not cheaper in dollars than nursing home care, does not prevent nursing home placement, and is certainly not cheaper in terms of the social and personal costs to the caregiver. Weissert concluded "The challenge . . . must be to find ways to finance . . . care for this new class of patients (that is, those who need long-term care), not to continue to try fruitlessly to justify community care as something it is not—a substitute for nursing home care or a way to save money" (p. 430). When institutional care is denigrated and the virtues of community care are extolled, the questions to be asked are "for whom?" and "compared to what?"

Though nursing home placement relieves some family strains, it does not end the family's long haul. Admission signals the beginning of a new phase in the family's odyssey, with some strains continuing and some new ones appearing. Though research on the family's experiences at this stage is meager, scattered findings mesh with copious clinical reports (Brody EM, 1981a). Many clinical reports describe the continuation of family concern, interest, and contacts with institutionalized older people. Family members often discuss the patient with nursing home personnel; they worry; they feel guilty at having placed their relative, no matter how clearly the harsh realities dictated that placement; they are sad at seeing the patient's continuing decline; and they experience depression and anxiety about their own aging. Family members may be upset about the quality of care and staff attitudes but are often in a bind—afraid to complain because they fear retaliation on the helpless resident, particularly when the afflicted person's cognitive state is such that he or she cannot report the things that happen.

Some of the family's distress may be related to a lack of clear role definition—ambiguity about the family's role vis-à-vis staff roles. Though the physical care of the disabled person (not specific to Alzheimer's disease) has been surrendered, how are roles as decision maker and care manager (for that is necessary in nursing homes no less than in the community) to be shared? Family members may be caught in a Catch-22: if they don't visit often, they are regarded by staff as unconcerned; if they do visit often, they may be viewed as nuisances.

There is little research specifically about the family relationships of institutionalized older people with dementia. The findings of one study, carried out at the Philadelphia Geriatric Center, indicates that such relationships remain important to both patients and their family members. It was found that demented women's emotional investment in their families had risen in relative importance between their middle years and old age (Kleban et al., 1971). Moreover, relationships of disabled persons with their families improve with psychosocial therapeutic intervention (Brody EM et al., 1971). The degree of cognitive impairment affected family visiting. Visits with deeply impaired relatives, although as frequent as to those with mildly demented patients, were shorter and less enjoyable to family members. Most of the relatives (70%) reported worrying about the Alzheimer patient and discussing him or her frequently with other family members (Moss & Kurland, 1979).

The study by George (1983) referred to above found no significant differences in mental health, stress symptoms, and physical health between caregivers whose relatives resided in long-term-care facilities and those caregivers whose afflicted relatives lived in the caregiver's household. When George (1984) followed-up the same families a year later, she found that caregivers who had placed the patient in a nursing home during the past year were more likely to be taking psychotropic drugs than were caregivers who cared for their relatives in the community or whose ailing relatives had died. Reports of stress symptoms and low levels of life satisfaction and emotional well-being were equal in those who had institutionalized the patient and those who were caring for the patient in their own home. In short, families of the institutionalized need help no less than families of community-dwelling patients.

The stresses of institutionalization are made all the more painful by the difficulties families have in locating a nursing home that will admit the patient, let alone one that provides quality care. Cost-containment policies now make it very difficult to effect admission of the "hard-to-care-for" Medicaid patient (U.S. GAO, 1984; Brody EM et al., 1984a), a phrase that often is a euphemism for the patient with Alzheimer's disease.

SUMMARY

In planning for the long haul, concentrated research that can prevent, cure, or ameliorate the emotional and social disruptiveness of Alzheimer's disease is a *sine qua non*. Until such a breakthrough occurs, it is necessary to alleviate strains on caregivers—not only by the provision of concrete in-home services and good nursing facilities, but also by means of counseling to help with the emotional stress that is so prevalent among families of Alzheimer patients (see also Tune et al., Chapter 7; Sainer, Chapter 11).

The best efforts of professionals and families can succeed only to the extent that social policy provides a context in which those efforts are fostered and supported and in which knowledge can be put into practice.

Current public policy is not helping ease the family's long haul. There has been virtually no social policy response to the needs of families (see also Williams, Chapter 9; Sainer, Chapter 11). For example, respite care and daycare are scarce and neither universally nor adequately available. There is limited regular public or private funding for their consistent support; programs that do exist are episodic, discontinuous, and vary greatly among the states (Meltzer, 1982). Economic supplements to caregiving families (e.g., attendance allowance, social security credits for caregivers remaining at home) are much more prevalent in other industrialized nations (Gibson MJ, 1984; see also Williams, Chapter 9). Community health and social services are limited and disproportionately under-financed as compared to acute medical care services for the aged (Brody SJ, 1979). Enormous inequities exist among the various states in their expenditures for Medicaid services, both for nursing home care and community-based services (e.g., see U.S. GAO, 1984). Inadequate reimbursement blocks access to quality nursing home care.

The role of professionals in gearing treatments to the long haul includes advocacy to see that society, through change in social policy, meets *its* responsiblities.

Grant support from The John A. Hartford Foundation and the Pew Foundation for a demonstration and research program at the Philadelphia Geriatric Center.

The author's own research was financed by NIMH grants   MH35252 and MH27361.

7
Psychosocial Interventions

*Larry E. Tune, Mary Jane Lucas-Blaustein, and
Barry W. Rovner*

The impact of Alzheimer's disease on victim and caregiver can be emotionally devastating. As the disease progresses over time, it produces disturbing cognitive, behavioral, affective, and physical symptoms. These can lead to a multiplicity of disruptions and disorders in those closest to the patient. Both patients and caregivers may need psychological support, beginning with the onset of cognitive impairment and continuing beyond the death of the patient, until the work of mourning has been completed.

Effective treatment depends on a trusting relationship among a team of professionals, the patient, and the caregivers. This is established early and maintained throughout the course of the disease. Family and close friends, who may serve as caregivers, provide the daily physical and emotional support for the patient. When they function as equal team members with professional staff in long-term planning and selection of options for the patient, they can most effectively supply the therapeutic environment needed by the patient. For the caregivers, Alzheimer's disease will affect relationships as well as mental and physical health. When the professional team provides support, information, resources, and training, caregivers can often fulfill their patient-care functions competently.

This chapter will explore psychological treatment strategies for the emotional issues that commonly emerge as Alzheimer's disease progresses. Such strategies can enhance the quality of life for both patient and family.

ESTABLISHING THE THERAPEUTIC RELATIONSHIP

We begin psychological treatment when patient and family first approach us (Steele et al., 1982). Even relatively mild early symptoms cause emotional distress to victims, close family, and friends. The patient may be frustrated by inexplicable lapses in mental function. Awareness of Alzheimer's disease and other forms of dementia may induce anxiety or denial with attempts to perform usual tasks as though nothing were wrong (see also Cohen, Chapter 5). Family and friends, too, may join the patient in denial and delay seeking help. As the cognitive impairment becomes more pervasive and interferes with most aspects of daily function, the deficits no longer can be minimized or denied and families seek help.

Diagnosis itself carries with it a prognosis of inevitable, progressive worsening and related symptoms. Lack of information may intensify anxiety and confusion among caregivers. Fear about possible hereditary tendencies may surface. Those closest to the Alzheimer patient may feel isolated and overwhelmed. Because the patient exhibits both abnormal and normal behaviors, caregivers experience confusion, anxiety, and frustration, which may be heightened by suggestions from other family members that those closest to the afflicted person are exaggerating the symptoms. Not uncommonly, symptoms are interpreted as intentional acts (on the part of the patient), performed to irritate and inconvenience the caregiver. Such misinterpretations and denial of the disease produce conflicting feelings and distorted perceptions, leading to strained relationships and intrapsychic distress.

Treatment begins with rigorous evaluation of the patient, family, and environment. As a part of the diagnostic process, we recommend a two-phase diagnostic conference, with sessions a few weeks apart. In the first session, questions and ventilation of feelings are encouraged in order to provide information and emotional relief for caregivers and to allow the professional staff to assess the emotional needs of the patient and family. The patient may be included in part of the discussion, depending on his or her clinical condition. If doubt and denial are strong, the family is encouraged to seek a second opinion. The first session may run anywhere from 30 minutes to two hours. The second session includes as many close family members and interested friends as possible and lays the groundwork for an enduring support network and trusting relationship between caregivers and professionals. The two-part diagnostic process allows caregivers to consult other professionals and to begin to plan concretely about their future. The second meeting is an opportunity for caregivers to ask detailed questions, to get information about specific resources, to deepen their understanding about the disease itself. They begin to function as part of a team, mapping long-term strategies for patient care. For the professionals these meetings provide the basis for a trusting relationship. They allow adequate assessment of the strengths and weaknesses of the support system and the identification of the most pressing therapeutic needs (Aronson & Lipkowitz, 1981; Bergmann et al., 1978; Johnson & Catalano, 1983; Ory et al., 1985)

THE THERAPEUTIC TEAM

The therapeutic team has five main functions: (1) providing counseling to caregivers as needed; (2) educating about the disease; (3) offering practical advice and referrals; (4) overseeing the psychological and medical treatment of the patient; and (5) training caregivers to function as at-home, on-the-spot case managers/therapists. The team takes an active stance, initiating discussion and making suggestions, is available in a consistent way over time, and maintains familiarity with the dynamics of each family. Composition of the psychotherapeutic team may vary, but often includes a physician, nurse, psychologist, and social worker. All professionals should be well trained in working with Alzheimer patients and caregivers. While each team member has some specific functions, most therapeutic tasks are assigned on the basis of logistics or relationship with specific patient or caregiver. The physician, for example, diagnoses, orders tests, prescribes medication, oversees physical aspects of treatment, and refers to other medical specialists as needed. The psychologist administers psychological tests, and the social worker serves as liaison with other service agencies. In our team, the nurse generally serves as co-therapist and coordinator of the management plan. Counseling, home evaluation, and education are shared by all members of the team. After the diagnostic conferences, the team assesses the immediate therapeutic issues for the patient and caregivers and assigns a primary therapist. The primary therapist meets with the caregivers and patient, takes a detailed psychological history, and is available, throughout the illness, for consultation and planned therapy sessions as needed. Suggestions for patient care tend to be received most favorably by caregivers when a solid relationship of trust and continuity has been established. To foster this relationship, we make our home phone numbers available to caregivers, so that they can consult the team at once if serious difficulties arise. Caregivers rarely abuse this accessibility.

EARLY CONFRONTATION OF LONG-TERM ISSUES

Planning and evaluation is an ongoing process that is continued during each regularly scheduled clinic visit, which occurs at roughly three-month intervals. To avoid crises, an effort is made to anticipate long-term psychological and social needs. At regular clinic visits, time is allotted not only for discussion of patient care but also for ventilation of feelings by caregivers. Caregivers are provided with specific information about Alzheimer's disease. Generally, such information arouses strong emotions; we acknowledge them and respond to them. The commitment of the professional team is itself therapeutic. It helps break down feelings of inadequacy and isolation that, if left unaddressed, could lead to exhaustion and feelings of helplessness in beleaguered caregivers.

Early education about available resources and concrete help in utilizing them is another aspect of emotional support. Caregivers are encouraged to investigate local Alzheimer support groups, adult daycare services, senior groups, and respite programs. Such resources may take months to mobilize, but awareness of their existence can make contact and utilization psychologically easier when the time comes for their use. Physical and occupational therapy, home repair and maintenance services, visiting nurses and transportation are also discussed in the early months of treatment. The order in which these areas are explored, and the relative weight attached to their discussion, varies from family to family, depending on the clinical situation (Mace & Rabins, 1982; Steele et al., 1982; Eisdorfer & Cohen, 1981; Reifler & Eisdorfer, 1980; Goldberg, 1981; see also Brody, Chapter 6; Reveley, Chapter 8; Sainer, Chapter 11).

Advice and referral for legal and financial matters are also part of our therapeutic plan. Early establishment of durable power of attorney is recommended, in order to avoid costly legal guardianship proceedings later on. Families frequently see this step as the stripping away of the patient's autonomy and dignity. Acknowledging caregivers' emotional and ethical conflicts helps family members make realistic decisions. A therapeutic environment where trust and forthrightness have been developed can make this painful task less difficult. When the patient is able to comprehend his or her situation adequately, we recommend presenting the proposal for durable power of attorney in these terms, "You know you have a memory problem; in case it gets worse it would be a good idea to have the person of your choice in charge of carrying out decisions you would want made." When the patient's cognition has slipped too far for meaningful participation, the family is asked to interpret the wishes and values of the patient and to develop a plan in accordance with them (see also Cassel & Goldstein, Chapter 4).

During the early months of treatment our team initiates discussion of nursing homes, though need for them may never materialize and is usually years away. Because the prospect of nursing home placement is so emotionally charged, we believe that it is best introduced long before its need is imminent. In such discussions family members are encouraged to ask questions and express feelings. Later the team suggests criteria according to which choices can be made and steers families away from inadequate homes. We encourage assessment of finances and recommend visits with nursing home staff. As practical steps are being encouraged, the staff also responds to the emotional issues that arise: fear of letting the afflicted person down; anticipated loss; guilt at being unable to continue with in-home care until the end. Providing opportunity for expression of feelings before the actual decision must be made clears the way for intelligent decision making, grounded in the realities of patient and caregiver needs and limitations. Caregivers are encouraged to think about the cutoff point, the conglomerate of circumstances under which maintaining home care is no longer viable (see also Reveley, Chapter 8).

Frequently families approach professionals with high hopes for medications to relieve symptoms. It is difficult for them to accept the limitations of medical interventions. We discuss the pros and cons of medication with caregivers throughout the course of the disease and pay attention to the despair that often underlies anxious questioning. While medications can alleviate many symptoms of Alzheimer's disease, families need help accepting that cognitive improvement is unlikely (see also Satlin & Cole, Chapter 3). Caregivers should be taught about adverse side effects (e.g., parkinsonian symptoms and excess sedation with neuroleptics). Caregiver observation can be of great use to the clinician in assessing the need for modifying medications.

TREATING THE ALZHEIMER PATIENT

Psychological treatment of the patient is a crucial element in comprehensive therapeutic planning. Occasionally a patient begins treatment in an early stage with such mild impairment that he or she has an acute and painful awareness of the changes that are starting to occur (see also Cohen, Chapter 5). For such patients, supportive therapy is possible. Grief and frustration over the losses already experienced and anticipatory grief over those to come are the major focal points in such therapy. Relational issues with spouse and other close family members may also be addressed. The patient is encouraged to ask questions and express feelings about the disease. Suggestions are made to the patient about practical measures he or she can take to compensate for cognitive losses, for example, making lists of tasks and the times they must be done, keeping schedules simple, always replacing objects in the same place (see also Winograd, Chapter 1; Burnside, Chapter 2). This direct treatment of the patient minimizes depression, anxiety, and disorientation in the early stages of the disease, and it can prolong independent functioning. Therapy is often offered directly by our staff (see also Cohen, Chapter 5), but most interventions are made by caregivers on an informal basis as they notice and respond to the emotional experience of the patient. Even when working with such mildly impaired patients, we do not delay the work with caregivers. Gradually, as the cognitive functioning of the patient declines, it is the caregivers who will take over major therapeutic as well as other caregiving functions. Early preparation can provide a gentler slope and avoid a rude shock for those close to a patient who was "doing so well" at the beginning of the treatment. Training caregivers to anticipate the patient's emotional needs and to respond with empathy and self-confidence is a priority of the health care team.

When the Alzheimer patient is severely amnestic (forgetful), the therapeutic concept of insight is no longer applicable. Such patients may still benefit from opportunities to express feelings as they arise. While professionals may participate in this process, it is usually those in daily contact with the patient who provide, in a supportive, nonconfrontational way, on-the-spot responsiveness, encouraging ventilation of feelings of loss, frustration, disappointment, and confusion.

Training caregivers to be empathic responders creates a foundation for the continuation of a satisfying and meaningful relationship between caregiver and patient for as long as possible. This training is the keystone in maximizing the emotional well-being of the Alzheimer patient.

There is no definite model of how to train caregiver-therapists, but commitment of the professional team to this idea is essential. Caregiver training takes place in an informal way during regular clinic visits. The professional asks about caregiver problems, for example, supervision and safety, mood disturbances, or behavioral symptoms. The professional inquires as to how the caregiver handles these problems and whether the outcome is satisfactory. If dissatisfaction is expressed, the professional may offer either insight about the underlying conflicts that may be preventing successful outcome or specific suggestions about possible caregiver interventions. For example, the professional might suggest that the caregiver verbally acknowledge the patient's frustration at growing incapacity.

As mentioned earlier, some caregivers believe that symptoms are under the control of the patient and represent the expression of antagonistic feelings. This belief creates a barrier to empathic response by the caregiver. Such a caregiver experiences the patient's forgetfulness as irresponsibility; disconnected remarks as attempts to embarrass; irascibility as lack of appreciation for the caregiver's efforts. The caregiver's own denial of the seriousness of the patient's illness makes it particularly difficult to accept the involuntary nature of the symptoms. Uneven progression of impairment adds to the difficulty. So, too, does the frequent phenomenon of the symptoms being exaggerated distillations of patient characteristics in his or her predisease state. One key element of training caregivers to be sensitive therapists for Alzheimer patients is to convince them that the symptoms are not voluntary. This is most fruitfully accomplished by having the patient attempt tasks in the presence of both professional and caregiver. For example, the professional may introduce him- or herself several times during an interview and then ask the patient to repeat back the name that was given. Demonstrating that the patient is unable to perform several such relatively simple tasks in a neutral context, uninfluenced by interpersonal conflicts between the patient and caregiver, is frequently persuasive. It may open the way for the professional to offer realistic suggestions to the caregiver.

Over time, with many such demonstrations and suggestions, the professional staff is able to convey to the caregivers a realistic assessment of the patient's capabilities and to teach the concept of shaping the environment to suit the needs of the patient. One significant benefit of this emphasis on training caregivers as primary therapists is that it is a process of empowerment in which caregivers, objectively caught in an increasingly demanding situation, can subjectively experience themselves as growing in competence and have that competence validated by the professional team.

No formal counseling can meet the daily emotional needs of the Alzheimer patient as well as can ongoing interventions by skilled caregivers. The goal in training caregivers is to teach them to provide a therapeutic environment in which many short, immediate interventions can be offered as needed.

Home evaluations, carried out periodically by the professional staff, provide further opportunities for training. During these home visits team members look for evidence of safety hazards, abuse, and physical or emotional problems. Explanations for troubling signs or symptoms are often discovered during such visits. For example, mysterious bruises on one patient were found to be the result of his walking into cactus plants in his beloved garden. The home visit provides a friendly occasion to make suggestions for psychological improvements and to validate the hard work, thoughtfulness, and creativity caregivers have exhibited.

EARLY AND MIDPHASE PROBLEMS OF CAREGIVERS

Caregiver problems progress as the duration of Alzheimer's disease lengthens (Zarit et al., 1980; Zarit & Zarit, 1982).

The Siege Mentality

Frequently, as symptoms worsen, caregivers develop a siege mentality, sacrificing much normal activity in order to attempt to gain control over the disease that now controls them (see also Brody, Chapter 6). Caregivers cannot easily acknowledge feelings of failure and frustration. To do so would be to face the basic losses they are experiencing: loss of control over their time, energy and money; loss of sleep; impairment of relationships; and, finally, the loss of a loved one, slowly, before their eyes. The siege mentality often obscures a mounting mood of anticipatory grief for the known person who is disappearing but who is at the same time so dramatically present. Caregivers caught up in these dynamics will not always ask for help. Yet when help is offered, it is rarely refused. In our experience, psychotherapists, if alert to it, can detect much underlying distress. When they closely monitor the caregiver's mental health, they may find that sometimes simply asking how things are going at home is enough to get the caregiver to open up. Sometimes further probing is required. The scheduling of "dead time" at each regularly scheduled clinical appointment allows us to do so. When stress is high and problems complex, we suggest that special appointments be set up. Such offers are usually accepted with eagerness. Ordinarily, a limited number of sessions is sufficient, though the same caregivers or families may need to repeat this series over the course of the disease.

Although lack of resources may force referral of caregivers with severe emotional distress out of the clinic for therapy, it is preferable, if possible, to provide needed counseling within the clinic in order to build on the comprehensive knowledge and trust accumulated over the long, shared ordeal of Alzheimer's disease.

Family Stress

Often the stress of Alzheimer's disease is destructive of family relationships. A 45-year-old woman, for example, with an afflicted mother and a 16-year-old son, may be exhausting herself providing adequate care for her mother, while neglecting her son, who begins to have problems in school. Or a wife may resent the financial and emotional resources her husband is devoting to his ailing father. When the locus of the Alzheimer-related strain is the family system itself, the whole family is encouraged to come for counseling. This is particularly true when longstanding marital tension that has gone unattended is submitted to the strain of Alzheimer's disease. The patient is often used as the scapegoat in such cases, in order to avoid confrontation of underlying dissatisfactions between the couple. Family therapy, or couple therapy, can take pressure off the patient. It is essential to note, however, that even good marital relationships may erode under the pressure of Alzheimer's disease.

It is of vital importance to give prompt and competent treatment to Alzheimer families in distress. Family turmoil creates a chaotic, hostile environment for the patient, which exacerbates the patient's symptoms and leads to an escalation of conflict in the family. It is wise to interrupt this disastrous spiral as early as possible. When family conflict is allowed to become severe, patients are often passed from one caregiver to another, or from one residence to another, in order to alleviate and redistribute the burdens. This denies the patient the very simplification and stability of environment needed to minimize excess disability. Such upheavals warrant intervention by the professional staff to convince the family to select one environment and make it work.

Shifting Roles

Family conflict is often precipitated by shifting roles, notably when the patient had formerly played a dominant role in the family. In traditional families, common among the current generation of elders, it is not unusual to find wives who do not drive and have never paid bills or taxes. When the wife is thrust into the role of caregiver to a husband suffering from Alzheimer's disease, acquiring necessary skills may impose excessive stress on an already stressed (and possibly aged and ailing) wife. Husbands, too, may have difficulty adapting to new demands made on them by having a wife with Alzheimer's disease, such as handling household management and providing emotional caregiving (see also Reveley, Chapter 8). Close monitoring of spouses undergoing role changes can decrease excess disability in the patient and mental and physical health problems in the spouse.

Group Therapy

Therapy and support groups can play an important role in moderating the overwhelming stresses brought on by Alzheimer's disease (Fuller et al., 1979). We encourage caregivers to join ongoing, therapist-led groups initiated by our clinic, as well as to become involved in organizations such as the Alzheimer's Disease and Related Disorders Association (see also Brody, Chapter 6; Reveley, Chapter 8; Sainer, Chapter 11).

We believe that ongoing, open-ended therapy can raise difficult issues and draw out feelings of anger and loss, creating a safe environment in which to take emotional risks. Group therapy is a natural treatment modality for people with shared problems. Groups provide a milieu in which the need for mutual dependence and feelings of unity can be expressed. Group cohesion permits emotional support to develop among people with mutual problems who can offer each other empathic understanding. Group problem solving offers solutions to practical problems. Reality testing, using the group for feedback, can have a powerful effect on people who have adopted myths and misconceptions about Alzheimer's disease. Finally, groups provide an opportunity to see that emotions often felt to be wrong or inappropriate are shared by others. Therapy groups can help caregivers feel better about an unyielding situation that itself cannot be changed.

MID- TO LATE-STAGE PROBLEMS FOR PATIENTS AND CAREGIVERS

Many of the psychological issues that emerge in earlier stages of Alzheimer's disease continue throughout the course of the illness, though prompt and appropriate interventions can mitigate their destructiveness and teach caregivers ways of coping that carry them through the long haul.

As the course of Alzheimer's disease continues, with increased deterioration in the patient, we have watched caregivers develop symptoms such as fatigue, depression, guilt, and a wish that the patient would die. Family stresses also tend to intensify.

The patient experiences the four A's of Alzheimer's disease. Progressive memory problems *(amnesia)*, loss of ability to understand or use language *(aphasia)*, loss of ability to perform voluntary motor tasks *(apraxia)*, and decline in ability to recognize objects *(agnosia)* are often accompanied by an increase in troublesome behavioral symptoms (e.g., wandering, aggressiveness, sleep disturbances). This places new demands on caregivers for supervision, patience, and understanding.

Educational work, begun in the early phases, must meet the new challenges. Demonstrating for caregivers the effects of each of the above-mentioned four A's of Alzheimer's disease helps caregivers understand the process of deterioration they are witnessing in the patient. Caregivers are helped to adapt to the reality that amnesia prevents the completion of tasks and can lead to the patient becoming lost; that aphasia may render the patient unable to articulate his or her wants or to participate in meaningful conversation; that an apraxic patient may have difficulty controlling machinery (e.g., an automobile) or feeding him- or herself; and that agnosia in its most disturbing manifestation may prevent the patient from recognizing loved ones. Explaining that lack of recognition of a particular caregiver does not mean lack of affection can lessen the pain felt by the unrecognized one. Unnecessary visits to medical specialists can also be averted through education: for example, agnostic patients often complain about their vision. Once evaluation has ruled out problems of visual acuity, knowledge of agnosia can prevent continued and futile visits to optometrists.

Physical violence, verbal abusiveness, suspiciousness, wandering, insomnia, eating disorders, and incontinence may stress caregivers beyond their endurance and raise the question of nursing home placement (see also Winograd, Chapter 1; Burnside, Chapter 2). Medications, when used with care, may help to alleviate behavioral manifestations. Maintaining environmental safety, simplicity, and stability for the patient, together with support and counseling for overwhelmed caregivers, can minimize the symptoms. Respite care can also alleviate some caregiver stress.

At the same time the professional team can help caregivers face the possibility that the time for placement in a nursing home is drawing near. When management of the patient becomes the central issue of family life and if it threatens to destroy the family, we usually recommend placement and facilitate its implementation (see also Burnside, Chapter 2; Cassel & Goldstein, Chapter 4; Brody, Chapter 6). Nursing home placement can reduce, if not resolve, marital and family issues, restore individual caregiver health, and remove the patient from the scapegoat position, allowing other family issues to be addressed.

END PHASE OF TREATMENT

The patient in the final stage is generally unaware of his or her specific surroundings and cannot appreciate or respond to caretakers in meaningful ways. The patient has become unable to participate in even simple social exchanges, to express basic needs, or to signify understanding when others try to communicate with him or her. Hence a profound separation between patient and family is common in the last stages of Alzheimer's disease.

Yet as impairment worsens, ever-increasing demands are placed on caregivers to feed, dress, bathe, and toilet the patient. These increased limitations and demands radically alter interpersonal family relationships, roles, and routines, placing caregivers at great risk for severe physical and emotional illness. Many caregivers are unable to accept the reality of the patient's condition and engage in a frustrating and futile attempt to maintain meaningful contact. Those caregivers who do resign themselves to the patient's limitations often suffer guilt feelings for having abandoned the loved one when they reduce frequency of visits (Niederehe & Fruge, 1984).

Caregiver treatment at this phase involves repeated acknowledgment of the stress under which the caregivers are living and of the magnitude of the impact of Alzheimer's disease upon their lives. Caregivers need reassurance that their responses are widely shared by others in similar situations. In the late stages of Alzheimer's disease, the existence of long-established relationships with professional staff and an ongoing therapy or support group can ameliorate the devastating effects of the disease on individual family members as well as family relationships (Rabins et al., 1982).

Prior exploration of nursing home facilities can greatly ease caregiver burdens in the final stages of Alzheimer's disease. While some patients (those fortunate to have generous financial resources and a healthy, willing spouse) remain in the home to the end, more often patients entering the vegetative condition can no longer receive adequate care at home (Wilder et al., 1983). In making recommendations we consider the health of the entire family as well as their financial, social, and emotional resources. If placement is necessary, our counseling focuses on separation anxiety, loss, and guilt; we assure the family that nursing home placement does not equal abandonment and that institutional life is not death. Many, though by no means enough, nursing homes are developing innovative programs to encourage continuing family participation in patient care.

It is in the end phase of Alzheimer's disease that ethical issues become most pressing. Dilemmas frequently arise about whether heroic measures should be taken to sustain life. Most families do not desire such measures, but many are reluctant to initiate discussion. Our professional team, therefore, opens discussion with caregivers, offering opportunity for ventilation of complicated and conflicted feelings about caregivers' own needs as well as their obligations to the patient (see also Cassell & Goldstein, Chapter 4).

Autopsy is another difficult issue, which we address when death approaches. Although it is painful for many families to authorize autopsy, we believe it is so important that it warrants discussion. Autopsy is the only means by which a definitive diagnosis of Alzheimer's disease can be made. At least one in 10 clinical diagnoses of Alzheimer's disease is found by autopsy to have been erroneous. Autopsy also provides needed tissue for research that may eventually provide a cure for the disease and allows for the charting of its genetic implications.

Finally, our observation suggests that the period of mourning following the death of the long-term Alzheimer patient may be relatively brief, possibly because anticipatory mourning has been going on for years. Nevertheless, there is often a surprising intensity to the grief experienced when the patient dies, even though the patient may have been in a vegetative state for years. Perhaps, when the need to contain emotion in order to carry on has been removed, the years of suffering and loss can at last be fully acknowledged and experienced. The continuing availability of the professional team and the support group can ease the grieving process for the survivors. While we have no formal program for long-term follow-up of such survivors, recognition of the impact of the disease on the whole caregiving network opens the way for understanding caregiving as a unique experience, with lasting consequences for individual caregivers and family systems. Professionals who are sensitive to the issues facing survivors can make known their accessibility for follow-up counseling as needed.

SUMMARY

Alzheimer's disease is a multifaceted process of deterioration, affecting the entire caregiving network as well as the patient. Early establishment of relationships of trust and cooperation between professionals (psychiatry, nursing, psychology, and social work), caregivers, and patients provides the basis for all further psychological treatment. Our professional team believes that an active, initiating stance by the professional staff is essential to good treatment. We offer practical help, including referrals to community resources, as well as emotional understanding, and try to ensure continuity and reliability of staff.

Unfortunately, neither professional training nor reimbursement policies foster the development of programs such as ours. Reimbursement based on a single treatment for a specific symptom on a given day runs counter to the realities of Alzheimer's disease and the needs of aged patients and caregivers. Clinical training and organization often fragment treatment, sending each patient and caregiver to a wide variety of specialists for treatment of this symptom or that, with little coordination or communication among the treating staff. Symptoms rather than persons are the subject of such treatment. We believe that an integrated long-term team approach, focusing on whole individuals and family relationships, is, in the long run, most effective and humane. It is our hope that reimbursement policy, professional training, and clinical organization will be reassessed to accommodate the real needs of Alzheimer patients and caregivers.

Grant support from: 1. Meridian Healthcare Systems; 2. Alzheimer's Disease Research Center NIA AG-05146; 3. Impact of Mental Morbidity on Nursing Home Experience NIA RO1 MH4 1570-4; 4. Barnes Fund; Dementia Research Clinic Gift Fund; Sandoz; American Foundation for Aging Research.

Acknowledgments: Ms. Karen Mullins for secretarial assistance.

8
One Caregiver's View

James B. Reveley

I might be the luckiest person alive. Lucky that is, within the context of being the caregiver for my wife, Priscilla, who was finally diagnosed as having Alzheimer's disease in 1980 and who was assuredly stricken at least two years before that.

First a bit about us. Priscilla is 63—young for her age and, except for Alzheimer's, in perfect health. She has been a schoolteacher, busy mother, and active volunteer worker, with special emphasis on her college, Bennington, in Vermont. Our son, Douglas, 36, is a chimney sweep and lives in New Hampshire with his 15-year-old daughter. His support and prayers, albeit across 400 miles, are crucial to our well-being. Our daughter, Elizabeth, 39, lives with her husband and 2-year-old daughter in Hawaii. She is a massage therapist and devotes volunteer time to massage therapy for Alzheimer's patients and canoe racers. When Priscilla's illness began, Elizabeth lived in Maine, was a watch officer at Outward Bound on Hurricane Island, and shared in the ownership and operation of a mussel farm. I am a retired banker. For 28 years I was in the field of trust and estate work and financial planning. For years I have grown exotic flowers under fluorescent lights, collected stamps, and puttered around the house. I am currently on the boards of four nonprofit organizations, specializing in finances and fundraising. I also was one of the three founders of the chapter of the Alzheimer's Disease and Related Disorders Association (ADRDA) in Rochester. To sum it up, I keep busy. It should also be noted before proceeding that we are atypical on two points: (1) I can financially handle all aspects of the disease, and (2) we brought to this ordeal an abiding love for each other.

The beginning was so uneventful and, as we exercise hindsight, so textbook; forgetting names, minimum confusion. Then one morning, two years later, I was sitting reading my breakfast-time newspaper. Priscilla asked me what I wanted for breakfast. I replied, "a poached egg." Some minutes passed and I sensed trouble. When I asked what was wrong, she turned to me with tears in her eyes and said, "What's a poached egg?" Moments later I had to go to work. What a day! Little was accomplished except making an appointment with Priscilla's general practitioner. He recommended a neurologist, who gave her a computed tomographic scan, electroencephalogram, and various standard evaluation tests. The verdict delivered by our doctor was Alzheimer's disease. He spent two sessions with me explaining and advising. Out of these sessions came two bits of advice which, learned in the beginning, were perhaps our salvation.

1. Do not hide the disease. Tell your friends and explain its symptoms and its course. Likewise, tell your children, but only face-to-face.
2. Live each day to the fullest, reach out to community resources, and maintain both your normal lives as long as possible. Most important, take care of yourself.

Within three weeks of the diagnosis, we had told most of our friends and had visited our children with the news. As luck would have it, Elizabeth talked about her mother's condition to the Outward Bound medical officer, who had recently received a form letter addressed to "Dear Colleague." It was from Boston's Beth Israel Hospital's Department of Neuropsychiatry, asking for volunteers for a lecithin study of Alzheimer's patients. On her next day off, Elizabeth was in Boston talking to the person in charge of the study about admitting Priscilla to it. Elizabeth was persuasive, and an interview was arranged for Priscilla. In spite of the distance from Rochester to Boston, Priscilla was accepted for a six-month study from January to July 1981. I also offered my services as a normal control person. And so we entered the mainstream of the Alzheimer's victim and caregiver.

Priscilla spent a week in the Clinical Research Center at Beth Israel having an intensive reevaluation and undergoing increasing lecithin dosage. I accompanied her to Boston and took many of the same tests she did. It was here we first learned of the staff's devotion to its participating families and the true worth of psychiatric social workers.

We returned home with Priscilla's lecithin mixtures and a challenge to make frequent trips to Boston for follow-up. Of the approximately 10 trips, Priscilla made six by herself. She was nervous and a bit unsure of herself. How to solve the problem?

I hit upon the idea of calling USAir's passenger agent in Boston and asked him for help. Together we arranged a plan that one of his agents would meet Priscilla's plane with a rose from me, present it to her, walk her to a taxi, and give the driver instructions to take her to Beth Israel. On the return, Beth Israel instructed the taxi driver to deliver her to USAir, who took over from there. How wonderful people are when called upon to help! This procedure was repeated five more times.

Even the IRS examiner who audited my 1981 return and found some taxi receipts missing, due to Priscilla's forgetting to procure them, cooperated and approved the taxi deduction.

In preparation for less happy times, I determined to learn about running a house. I was now on Priscilla's home turf, and learning and practicing was not easy. Today I can clean, wash, and iron, and I consider myself somewhat of a gourmet cook. Alas, I have never learned hand sewing nor probably ever will. My best time threading a needle is 90 seconds. Need I go further?

I also found support services rather minimal for Alzheimer families in Rochester—so with two wonderful women I founded ADRDA–Rochester. Our chapter provides the caregiver information about the disease, availability of community services, nursing homes, and legal and financial advice. We also provide speakers and general information to the community at large. Political advocacy on the local level and awarding of modest sums for local research complete our programs. Our ADRDA chapter is now administering to over 200 families and since June 1984 has had a full-time office in the Neuropsychiatry Offices at the University of Rochester, Strong Memorial Hospital.

In midsummer 1981, Priscilla and I agreed to participate in the TV show "Someone I Once Knew." This is a one-hour documentary program produced by Channel 5 in Boston. It describes for the layperson Alzheimer's disease as seen through researchers' and clinicians' eyes. Interwoven throughout are interviews with several victims and their caregivers. We were invaded by a friendly crew of five to produce many hours of tapes, in both Rochester and Boston. Edited, it resulted in perhaps 10 minutes of the program. It was a hilarious experience and could provide another whole paper. One amusing incident was picking up the Sunday *Times* over and over while riding our bicycles until the director felt the scene played right. Then the whole episode wound up on the cutting room floor.

Summer turned to fall, and we continued our crusade through radio and TV vignettes and speaking to local civic and religious groups. The name Alzheimer's disease slowly but surely was becoming known.

The months turned into years, and Priscilla has slid down the scale of full mental competency. In 1983 we moved our case to the Alzheimer's Clinic in Rochester and again Priscilla entered a drug trial program and I joined a normal control person group. We have been CATted and PET-ted and NMRed and psychologically tested. One time I was doing mazes and the tester was excited because I was about to solve a difficult one. You all know the two rules about maze testing—you can't backtrack and you can't take your pencil off the paper. Well, suddenly both my nose and fanny started to itch simultaneously. So now you know how I came out on the test.

At about this time Priscilla began speech therapy. Her therapist is a remarkable woman and has been able to keep Priscilla communicating at a rather high level.

Our children have been wonderful. Calls, letters, pictures, and visits to see them and our grandchildren abound. And it's not hard to spend a couple of weeks a year visiting family in Hawaii, we just returned. Last Christmas I gave my son, daughter, and myself TV cameras and VCRs, so now we really communicate. What wonders technology can accomplish to hold far-flung families together.

We also bought a dog—an eight-week old white standard poodle—now 2 years old and full grown at 55 pounds. How lucky can you get—we both love him. Priscilla remembers his name, his sex, when and what to feed him, and when to exercise him. I groom and bathe him and do some walking.

Our friendships are evolving. Acquaintances have dropped off, but dear friends remain and new ones are added. We go out at least once a week and could go twice. I have neighborhood friends who monitor Priscilla's walks and are available to sit by the hour or the day. I have volunteers who, for modest pay, will sit for 24 hours or longer. I am still working to expand this area. Old friends from all over the world have become pen pals.

Our support network is growing—some volunteered and some joined merely by my asking. Let me give you a few examples:

My former employer and fellow workers. I can't say enough for all of them. Before I retired, time off was never a problem and their personal support during the five years I worked for them while I was a caregiver was super. Even after my retirement they gave financial support to ADRDA, and their word-processing unit has typed this chapter. Super people, all of them.

Clothing. I called the president of a local department store for shopping advice and assistance. I now have assigned to us a delightful woman who assists me by phone and in visits to the store. She has also stated that someone would come to the house with selections if and when necessary.

Hairdresser and manicurist. Both are showing me how to help on repairs and redos between visits. Both will make house calls at no extra charge when worse comes to worse because of their high regard for Priscilla.

Dry cleaner. They will do all my sewing and repair and button replacement. A seamstress has even offered to come to the house—at an additional charge, of course.

My church. This is the most difficult area I and others have encountered. Upon querying other caregivers and several priests and rabbis, I found neither side was comfortable with the situation. Basically, it revolved around two intertwining problems. First, what does the caregiver want from his church or temple and second, how does the priest or rabbi approach the family. We have not found all the answers, but ADRDA–Rochester has held its first seminar for ministers, priests, and rabbis and we are making progress.

Legal work and financial planning. I got our lawyer interested and, between him and me (remember, I was a financial planner), we have designed excellent wills. In the process our lawyer has become an expert in the field of shielding assets for people and families with long-term illnesses. We have also signed our living wills and organ-donor cards.

Food tasters. Two couples have volunteered to taste test my cooking—gourmet or otherwise. If I pass, we go on to dinners of three and four couples. If I flunk—well, as they say, back to the drawing board.

Long ago and far away. Priscilla has a high level of recall for events in the 40's and 50's. As a teenager she was an accomplished horsewoman who showed other persons' horses in and around Litchfield, Connecticut, and later in Madison Square Garden in New York City. However, she had not ridden in over 40 years. As luck would have it, this summer I met an 83-year-old retired Army cavalry officer who has two horses and is somewhat knowledgeable about Alzheimer's disease. Working over a month from simply patting the horses to mounting, Priscilla is now riding by herself in a ring. We will not permit her to jump, but she is ever so happy. And that's what it's all about.

We try to keep up a normal life and laugh and love and go to sleep each night in each other's arms. Most important, so far I am managing to maintain Priscilla's dignity. Our goal is two successes a day—no matter how trivial. For example: we got dinner for six on the table all in the proper sequence and at the proper temperature; Sam, our dog, performed all his obedience work perfectly and he gave us both kisses; I learned we had successfully reached our fundraising goal for our local ADRDA chapter.

For the real future, I have toured two nursing homes—as it happens, both are nonprofit, church-affiliated ones. Both are excellent, but I have not yet put Priscilla's name on the waiting list. That can wait until the time comes. "When the time comes," what a glib phrase. How will I know when that is? There are no set answers, only guidelines. But let me try anyway. Priscilla, because she is in an ongoing program, is evaluated rather often by a neuropsychiatrist. I encourage him to be frank with any assessment that must then trigger action on my part. In the calmness of this moment my triggers will be based on three criteria:

> I know in my heart that better care can be provided to Priscilla by a nursing home than I can provide in our own home;
> A sudden change might come making it clear even to myself that I can no longer manage;
> I know that I am caring for Priscilla at home, not for her sake, but for mine, under a misguided sense of duty that will only bring disaster to both of us and our family.

Can I abide by these criteria? There is only one answer. I must.

Another word about me. Late last fall an accumulation of things led me to a psychiatric counselor for help. She was wonderful. She got me back on course in about six weeks. Then near-disaster struck. A physical exam plus a treadmill stress test suggested a heart problem. Two weeks later a thallium stress test showed negative, so all is again well with this caregiver. But it did show a glaring hole in my plans: let's face it, I might be the first to die. I am still working on this problem and am making some progress, but I have no solution yet.

Let me summarize:

- Don't hide the disease
- Enlist help in all areas—people are wonderful
- Take calculated risks (such as Priscilla's going alone to Boston)
- Check wills and finances
- Enjoy life as long as possible
- Where available, join in the medical–psychiatric support system— it's a savior
- Maintain the dignity of your spouse and love, love, love

I can't end this paper without a tribute to the many professional helpers and what they represent. I want you to know that keeps us going.

To the social workers, I want to say that you and your profession help us all so much. As you go home at night exhausted and near burnout, remember, our days are made easier because of your efforts.

To all researchers and gerontologists, I want to tell you to keep up the good work. The answers will come. If not in time for us, then for those who follow.

And finally, I must end with a tribute to my wife, Priscilla. A fighter when the odds are totally against her—a winner while losing. Still with so much awareness that she thanks me for being her husband and caregiver. Can you imagine that!

Bless you all. You give true meaning to the phrase, "You do not walk alone."

POSTSCRIPT

Time goes on—some of it good, some not so good. I have become totally goal and project oriented in timeframes ranging from the next hour to the coming year. It gives me a tomorrow, and Priscilla seems to thrive on it.

For example: *Christmas and its preparation.* The two of us, with no assistance, held our 47th annual (started by my parents and taken over by us in 1952) Christmas Eve open house for 60 old friends—aged 2 to 85. Two years ago I took videocassette pictures of the dressing of the house, Christmas tree, and table tops, and the arrangement of the "festive board." We vied with each other to recreate everything as it has been for many years. Priscilla can no longer bake, so I made the cookies and breads while she greased pans and cleaned up. Years of tradition and memories paid off; the party was a smashing success! Christmas Day we were invited for dinner at the home of dear friends, who bent over backwards to make it perfect for us.

January has been spent making plans for a February visit from our son. Simultaneously, we are beginning preparations for a surprise 40th birthday party for our daughter Elizabeth, to be held in Hawaii. Our first action is to assemble, mount, and label a photo album and scrapbook of her 40 years. Bringing order out of the chaos of mountains of unidentified, jumbled-up photos has been a challenge, and Priscilla has joined in enthusiastically (if not always helpfully). We have been so successful, with fun for me and recall for her, we are now starting on one for our son, Douglas, and a combined one of the two of us since birth. It can and will be useful as memory fades.

We go everywhere. Priscilla has maintained a high degree of the social graces, so she is a joy to be with, a view shared by me and her many friends, who still take her to meetings and luncheons. And equally important, thanks to speech therapy she can make herself understood.

And what of the future? While we can, we are going to enjoy ourselves, even as Priscilla slowly slips into darkness. We have plans for the rest of the year, and for sure we will be in Hawaii in October for Elizabeth's party. I will continue in my work with the local and state Alzheimer's organizations, hoping always that the next generation will perhaps know a cure and benefit from our experiences.

In our own small way, we intend to leave our mark. And now to get on with it! There's much to be done, times to enjoy, and love to share. And who knows how much time for it all?

PART III
Policy

9
Public Policy Issues

T. Franklin Williams and Barbara Katzman

There is no question that Alzheimer's disease will be a major issue for health care providers and public policymakers for years to come. The real question is whether the future is an optimistic one, including precise diagnostic capabilities and reliable treatment and prevention, or a clouded one, as predicted by Dr. Edward Schneider, deputy director of the National Institute on Aging: "As progress continues against cardiovascular disorders and cancer, Alzheimer's disease will emerge as the leading cause of death for Americans in the 21st century" (Eckholm, 1985).

As the number of persons aged 65 years and older increases, so too does the number of those suffering from Alzheimer's disease; hence the ever-increasing need for a viable long-term health care policy. Given the complexities of the problem, where should policy priorities be placed? In this chapter we will consider four policy-related issues: financial considerations, research, options for care, and training. These issues have been carefully assessed by the Alzheimer's Disease Task Force (U.S. Department of Health and Human Services, 1984a) appointed by the Secretary of the Department of Health and Human Services, and discussed more fully in their report.

FINANCIAL CONSIDERATIONS

According to the American Association of Retired Persons, nearly 80% of older people in this country believe that their insurance is adequate to cover catastrophic illness (Quinn, 1985). In truth, most older people and their families are ill-prepared to deal with the costs of a major chronic illness.

147

Surveys of older people in Massachusetts show that two-thirds of persons 66 years of age and older who are living alone would become impoverished after only 13 weeks in a nursing home. Thirty-seven percent of married couples in that age group would become destitute within 13 weeks if one spouse required nursing home care (House Select Committee on Aging, 1985). A study conducted at the National Institute on Aging estimates that expenses incurred by caring for an Alzheimer patient at home are equally prohibitive: total per patient expenditures of direct and indirect costs amounted to a staggering $11,735 per year (Huang et al., 1988). Considering the fact that the average life expectancy of an Alzheimer patient is 8 years from diagnosis (see also Winograd, Chapter 1) and that many victims live quite a bit longer, nursing home care usually becomes necessary during the course of the disease. Current public and private insurance programs are not likely to protect the older individual from monumental health care costs. A special recommendation was made for financial relief in Alzheimer cases by the Report of the Secretary's Task Force on Alzheimer's Disease (U.S. Department of Health and Human Services, 1984a).

What steps have been taken by policymakers to help meet these burgeoning health care costs of Alzheimer's disease patients and their families? Over the past few years, several bills have been introduced in Congress to attempt to find financial solutions to this difficult problem. The enactment of the Alzheimer's Disease and Related Dementias Services Research Act of 1986 (Title IX, PL 99-660), passed by Congress and signed by the President, is a landmark piece of legislation insofar as it addresses the tremendous scope of the problem. The law emphasizes the need to learn more about the dementias affecting predominantly older persons and the importance of both formal and informal support systems to assist families in care management. Further, it reflects an understanding of the tremendous cost that families incur as a result of this illness.

The act establishes a Council on Alzheimer's Disease whose mission is to: (1) coordinate continuing research, (2) establish a mechanism for sharing information with health care providers of older people, (3) identify the most promising areas of research, (4) establish mechanisms so that research findings can influence policies and programs in order to improve the quality of life for older Americans, and (5) assist the National Institute on Aging, the National Institute of Mental Health, and the National Center for Health Services Research and Health Care Technology Assessment in developing and coordinating the research required to comply with this law. Additionally, the act established an advisory panel to identify for the Council priorities and emerging issues in the care of individuals suffering from dementia. As specifically stated in this provision, the panel is to apprise the Council of innovative methods of financing health care and social services for Alzheimer's disease patients and families. Further provisions of this legislation are presented in the section on research.

President Reagan, Secretary of Health and Human Services Dr. Otis R. Bowen, and members of Congress have given a great deal of time and thought to the enactment of a catastrophic health care bill to ease the financial burdens of major illnesses. Toward this end, the House of Representatives recently passed, and the Senate is considering, legislation that would provide catastrophic health insurance for Medicare beneficiaries. However, neither long-term health care nor long-term nursing home care is covered in this bill.

Proposals have been introduced in Congress to either expand Medicare to cover additional payment for the long-term cost of Alzheimer's disease or to find innovative ways to protect families from the high costs of home health care. For example, Representative Edward R. Roybal (D-Calif.), Chairman, House Select Committee on Aging, in 1987 introduced a bill entitled the Comprehensive Alzheimer's Assistance, Research, and Education Act (CARE) (HR 3130). The bill would provide, among other things, expanded family support and service delivery, money with which to provide families with community in-home care services, legal counseling, education, and respite care. Other bills have been proposed as well. An amendment to the Internal Revenue Code of 1986 (HR 631) was introduced in 1987 by Representative Silvio Conte (R-Mass.). This provision would entitle families caring for relatives with Alzheimer's disease to an income tax credit. The Alzheimer's Disease and Related Dementias Home and Community-Based Services Block Grant of 1987 (S 81) was introduced by Senator Howard Metzenbaum (D-Ohio). The purpose of this bill is to guarantee that certain in-home and community-based services such as respite care, training and counseling for family members, personal homemaker services, transportation, and hospice care are available to those who could benefit from them. This legislative activity reflects the wide range and extent of Congressional interest in Alzheimer's disease.

The Health Care Financing Administration (HCFA), the agency that manages Medicare and Medicaid, is actively involved in exploring ways to make medical benefits fiscally sound and more responsive to the needs of long-term care recipients. As a result of the Tax Equity and Fiscal Responsibility Act (TEFRA) of 1982 (PL 97-248), group practice organizations, such as health maintenance organizations (HMOs) and independent practice associations (IPAs), may now provide health care for Medicare recipients through a prepayment plan as an alternative to fee-for-service. Two obvious benefits reaped from such an arrangement are that medical expenses can be budgeted and that there are no additional out-of-pocket costs to members. A new addition to this system, being tested in several demonstration projects, is the inclusion of social service benefits and long-term care coverage (S/HMO) for prefixed payments (Davis, 1985). These relatively new plans must be evaluated for effectiveness of service delivery, quality of care, and financial viability, particularly for individuals and families faced with the long-term burdens of Alzheimer's disease.

Several large private insurance companies offer policies that pay for in-home health care services. Assistance in housekeeping tasks, shopping and cooking chores, and personal hygiene are included in these policies. Some insurance companies cover nursing home care as well. However, many older people on fixed incomes cannot afford the insurance policies offered by the corporate sector.

Solutions must be found to ease this difficult and complex problem of providing affordable yet comprehensive health care coverage to all people.

RESEARCH

A second general priority area emphasized in the Report of the Secretary's Task Force on Alzheimer's Disease (U.S. Department of Health and Human Services, 1984a) is that of research. The report lists nine main areas of research relevant to Alzheimer's disease: epidemiology, etiology, pathogenesis, diagnosis, clinical course, treatment, family involvement, systems of care, and an emphasis on training clinical personnel and releasing educational materials and information to professionals and the public. These nine areas cover a spectrum from basic research to information dissemination.

The Alzheimer's Disease and Related Dementias Services Research Act, referred to earlier, is a sign that research on the dementias has been given a high priority by Congress. It directs the National Institute on Aging, the National Institute of Mental Health, the National Center for Health Services Research and Health Care Technology Assessment, and the Health Care Financing Administration to conduct and support research on Alzheimer's disease. It also directs the National Institute on Aging to establish a clearinghouse to ensure that research advances are accessible to those individuals and families who would benefit most. It is anticipated that this information center will be fully operational in 1988.

Earlier Congressional actions have included directives to the National Institute on Aging to establish ten Alzheimer's Disease Research Centers (ADRCs) to conduct basic and clinical research and to disseminate research findings. Congress has also directed the establishment of a network of Alzheimer's disease case registries to enable additional epidemiologic research on the nature and cause of the disease. These programs are proceeding vigorously.

Investigators across the country and the world are devoting their time and effort into finding causes, treatment protocols, and possible cures. During the Differential Diagnosis of Dementing Diseases Consensus Conference held at the National Institutes of Health (U.S. Department of Health and Human Services, 1987a) researchers from around the country attempted to determine the most precise methods of diagnosing Alzheimer's disease. The basic conclusion of the conference was that further studies are vitally necessary to be able to reliably diagnose and predict dementia of all types. Every patient with dementia deserves precise assessment, not only of the presence of dementia, but of the manifestations and the manner in which the disability is produced. Priorities for the future, as established by the panel, are the exploration of potential biological diagnostic markers and the evaluation of neuroimaging through long-term follow-up of patients.

Current research advances in understanding the basic nature of Alzheimer's disease, its causes, course, and possibility for prevention and treatment are discussed in Chapter 13. In 1986, the total annual Federal support for research on Alzheimer's disease was approximately $61 million of which the National Institute on Aging provided 54 percent; the National Institute of Neurological and Communicative Disorders and Stroke, 25%; the National Institute of Mental Health, 15%; and the Veterans Administration, 4%. Even though this research support is seemingly impressive, in fact, it is equivalent to less than $\frac{2}{10}$ of 1% of the estimated $38 billion in direct costs spent on this disease annually (Huang et al. 1988).

Internationally, the Secretary's Task Force on Alzheimer's Disease has recommended the initiation of international studies to expand our understanding of Alzheimer's disease. Among its activities, the National Institute on Aging has a key role in helping to develop the World Health Organization's Special Programme for Research on Aging. A priority research area of this program is to conduct studies of dementia in various world populations. In addition to the WHO initiative, the Pan American Health Organization is launching a study on Alzheimer's disease as well. A recent forum on dementia held in Italy further demonstrates the worldwide concern over this devastating disease. From comparative studies with other countries and other cultures, we can hope to discover clues to the cause(s) of this disease and innovative ways of developing quality care.

OPTIONS FOR CARE

Alzheimer's disease has far-reaching medical, psychological, social, and economic implications. We need to stand back, perhaps, to gain a clearer perspective of the problems and their potential solutions. One step in this process should be a thorough assessment of both the immediate and long-term needs of the patient and the family. Physicians, nurses, and social workers trained in geriatrics can help identify previously un-recognized problems and develop a therapeutic plan tailored to each situation. Public policy must help ensure that such comprehensive assess-ment and care management services are available, as has been developed in several demonstration projects; see, for example, the ACCESS pro-gram in Rochester, New York (Eggert & Brodows, 1982) (see also Winograd, Chapter 1; Burnside, Chapter 2; Cohen, Chapter 5; Brody, Chapter 6; Tune et al., Chapter 7; Sainer, Chapter 11).

During the initial stages of Alzheimer's disease, afflicted individuals are generally able to function with minimal external aid. As the disease progresses, however, help is often required for housekeeping and per-sonal hygiene. Late stages of the disease often make nursing home care essential. Based on a thorough evaluation of need, a full range of options should be considered. Public policy also must consider and develop ways to provide these options of care:

Home Support Services are crucial in allowing patients to remain as independent as they are capable of being. Some may need assistance for accomplishing everyday tasks, others for transportation, still others for physical therapy. A good system of home support services will provide the individual with just the amount of care necessary—no more, no less—in this way fostering continued independence rather than depen-dence (Brody EM, 1977).

Adult Day Programs provide supervision, social activities, and meals, and rehabilitative therapies, such as physical and occupational therapy, should be available. Such programs enable caregivers to contin-ue their own jobs and/or have relief from the responsibilities of caregiv-ing for a portion of one or more days a week. This eases to some extent the tremendous personal and financial burdens which may be placed upon the caregiver.

Respite Care provides temporary care to Alzheimer patients and other severely impaired adults, either within the patient's home, or through temporary admission to a nursing home. This gives the family some planned time away from the grueling responsibility of caring for a severely ill relative.

Nursing Home and Supervised Residential Care Programs are geared to the special needs of Alzheimer victims, and should be available for seriously afflicted persons who do not have adequate family support or whose needs have exhausted such supports. Inasmuch as many Alzheimer patients continue to be in good physical condition even when quite confused and forgetful, the environment of such facilities should provide protected areas, indoors and outdoors, for walking without risk of wandering off, and should offer regular, familiar daily activities tailored to individual preferences. The Department of Health and Human Services has proposed more stringent regulations for round-the-clock quality of care for nursing homes.

TRAINING

Another policy issue is that of adequate training of professionals. There is an obvious shortage of trained professionals who are capable of caring for Alzheimer patients and who understand the special needs they impose. The need for increased training programs at all care levels cannot be overstated.

Two recent Department of Health and Human Services reports recommend increased training and education in geriatrics and gerontology by expanding existing programs and instituting new ones (U.S. Dept. of Health and Human Services, 1984c, 1987b). The earlier report states that, though progress is being realized, the shortage of physicians, nurses, and social workers trained in geriatrics will continue to pose a problem to the growing number of older people. More researchers in the field of aging also are vitally necessary if we are to improve the quality of life for our older population. In a more recent report required by Congress, the Department reported on the personnel needs for caring for older people. High priority was given to training well-educated health personnel ranging from aides to medical specialists.

The National Institute on Aging has initiated several approaches to fulfill these needs. The most current of these is the Leadership and Excellence in Alzheimer's Disease (LEAD) Award, recently authorized by Congress (PL 99-660). This is an award to stimulate high quality research by encouraging investigators who have already made significant contributions to Alzheimer's disease research to commit their time exclusively to this area. Recipients of the award are expected to enlist the assistance of promising junior researchers to strengthen and expand the nucleus of people who can make significant progress in this field.

CONCLUSION

The cost of caring for Alzheimer patients in the United States is estimated to be more than $38 billion per year, an amount that shows every indication of increasing substantially over the next several years (Huang et al., 1988). The ultimate answer to this epidemic must come from research, pursued as vigorously as we have pursued other scourges such as tuberculosis, cancer, and, more recently, acquired immune deficiency syndrome (AIDS). Meanwhile we need well-defined, cohesive approaches to care in which both clients and those who finance services (public or private) can feel confident.

The opinions expressed herein are those of the author and not necessarily those of the Federal Government.

10
The Role of the Veterans Administration

Edwin J. Olsen, John H. Mather, James L. Fozard, and Alan M. Kennedy

The Veterans Administration's (VA) role in long-term care of veterans with dementia is influenced by several basic factors: (1) eligibility for VA care, (2) demographics of the veteran population, (3) prevalence of dementia, (4) family responsibilities and pressures, and (5) social and medical care systems.

The VA's programs for demented patients include education, research, and patient-enhancement activities. For both demented and nondemented, the VA operates 172 hospitals, 226 outpatient clinics, 119 nursing homes, and 16 domiciliary care units. (Domiciliary care provides residential and medical care to ambulatory veterans who do not require hospitalization or skilled service of a nursing home.) In addition, the VA assists states in operating 50 state Veterans' Homes (thus providing direct hospital, nursing home, and domiciliary care under the auspices of individual states) plus three state Home Annexes in 35 states; it also contracts with approximately 3,200 community nursing homes to provide veterans with limited-term posthospital care. All of these facilities are potential sites for the care of veterans with dementia, depending on the level of care needed. There are, however, eligibility criteria that limit which veterans may be admitted for care.

ELIGIBILITY

Under Title 38 of the U.S. Code, the VA must give first priority to providing health care to veterans with service-connected disabilities—wounds or medical conditions incurred during active military service. For the great majority of veterans, dementia is diagnosed long after discharge from active service and is, therefore, considered a nonservice-connected disability. For veterans with a service-connected disability who also have dementia, his or her right to priority for admission and the period of stay in a Veterans Administration Medial Center would be determined by the treatment needs for the service-connected disability rather than for the dementia.

Public Law 99-272, signed into law on April 7, 1986, made several changes in veterans' eligibility for VA health care. The intent of the law is to ensure that VA hospital care is available to low-income veterans as well as to veterans with service-connected disabilities (disabilities incurred in or aggravated by active military service). Veterans with higher incomes will be provided VA health care on a space-available basis and may be charged a deductible for their care based on their level of income.

Exceptions to the new, income-based eligibility assessment include:

- veterans with service-connected disabilities
- former prisoners of war
- veterans exposed to herbicides in Vietnam or to ionizing radiation during atmospheric testing and in the occupation of Hiroshima and Nagasaki who need treatment for a condition that might be related to the exposure
- veterans receiving a VA pension
- veterans of the Spanish-American War, the Mexican border period, or World War I
- veterans eligible for Medicaid

The new eligibility assessment applies to all other veterans with nonservice-connected disabilities, regardless of age.

The veteran with nonservice-connected dementia who has a concurrent illness requiring immediate hospital treatment will be admitted for the duration of that acute episode if a bed is available. However, a veteran with nonservice-connected dementia alone may have difficulty gaining admission to a VA hospital. Admission decisions are made by clinicians at each hospital, based on their evaluation of the need and the resources available. Cognitive impairment alone may not be considered a medical reason for an acute admission to a hospital.

For veterans who are already in the VA system, the recent application of new guidelines for the use of staff and other resources leads to reevaluation of the appropriateness of continued hospital or nursing home care. A veteran with dementia who is ambulatory and does not need 24-hour nursing care, for instance, may be recommended for transfer out of a nursing home to his own home or another noninstitutional mode of care. A veteran who has been hospitalized in a VA's intermediate care unit may be determined not to require hospital care and be transferred to a nursing home. If a VA nursing home bed is not available, a transitional stay in a private or nonprofit nursing home is arranged, but this is limited to six months at VA expense for veterans with nonservice-connected disabilities. After six months, the veteran's family is required to provide home or nursing home care at their own expense unless they are eligible for Medicaid. The requirement for Medicaid eligibility is that the veteran and usually his spouse must be "medically indigent," that is, to have spent all of their savings and in some states to have sold their property.

DEMOGRAPHICS OF THE VETERAN POPULATION

America's aging veterans continue to represent an increasing proportion of the older population. Because of the large number of men and women who served the country in World War II and the Korean War, this group of Americans has a unique age distribution. Compared to the general population, a higher proportion of this group is over 65 years of age, and this proportion is growing—from 10.5% in 1980 to 37% projected by the year 2000 (U.S. Veterans Administration, 1984). This 37% subgroup of veterans over 65 will compare to only 13% in that age group in the general population.

This means that an increasing proportion of America's elderly are veterans and may be calling upon the VA for care. They will be subject to an increasing incidence of illness and infirmity, including dementia, which will require long-term care. Consequently, the VA has been planning for the large increases in the geriatric subgroup who will seek care from the VA's Department of Medicine and Surgery. These preparations include significant improvements and innovative approaches in three of the missions for which the Department is responsible—patient care, education, and research.

PREVALENCE OF DEMENTIA

Dementia is a chronic illness that becomes more prevalent with advanced age. Dr. James A. Mortimer, epidemiologist at the VA Medical Center's

Geriatric Research, Education and Clinical Center (GRECC) in Minneapolis, has estimated that at the present time 1.2 million individuals in the United States aged 65 and over have dementia (Mortimer et al., 1981). Based on data from Kay and colleagues (1970) and Hagnell and colleagues (1981), Mortimer estimates that more than 200,000 veterans were afflicted by severe dementia in 1980 and that this prevalence will more than double (to over 500,000) by the year 2000. Incidence, he predicts, will triple over these same decades from approximately 25,000 new cases in 1980 to 75,000 in the year 2000. With the growing proportion of elderly who are veterans, this rise in incidence may make great demands upon the resources of VA facilities.

Information from the VA's computer database bears out Mortimer's prediction of a sharply rising trend. The number of VA hospital discharges with a primary diagnosis of dementia increased at a rate of over 12% a year from FY 1981 to FY 1984—an overall increase of 47% in four years. The increase was observed in virtually every diagnostic classification for dementia. This probably represents a greater awareness and an improved diagnostic acumen vis-à-vis dementia. The VA estimates that 11,200 veterans were treated for dementia as a primary diagnosis in FY 1984. Based on discharge and inpatient census data, if the second through fifth diagnosis recorded on the patient's charts were included, this number would exceed 20,000. Given Mortimer's estimate of 200,000 veterans with severe dementia in the early 1980s, this estimate of 20,000 appears small. This means that the VA is providing care for probably only 10% of the veterans with severe dementia. A very large pool of potential patients are either not eligible or are receiving care elsewhere and are not currently seeking medical care through the VA.

FAMILY RESPONSIBILITIES AND REACTIONS

As in the private sector, the VA's role in the care of patients with dementia is influenced by the extraordinary emotional and physical burdens that are experienced by family members. Those families providing care at home—particularly if they attempt to undertake this alone, without advice, respite, or other support (Zarit & Zarit, 1982)—may eventually become exhausted or ill and feel unable to go on. The veteran patient may then be brought to the VA's doorstep with an urgent plea for inpatient care. Families often report that it is not easy to find a VA medical center near their homes that will admit a veteran whose primary complaint is dementia, thus experiencing the same frustrations, bewilderment, fear, and anger as families seeking care in other sectors of the health care system.

The growing recognition of dementing illness as a major public health problem that places financial and other burdens on the family has led to the formation of advocacy and family support groups, often combined, such as the Alzheimer's Disease and Related Disorders Association (ADRDA). The VA encourages the formation of family and caregiver support groups, although it may have no formal relationship to them.

SOCIAL AND MEDICAL CARE SYSTEMS

U.S. social and medical structures do not always provide options to care for individuals who are demented. As with the population in general, veteran patients and families are frequently faced with the alternatives of providing (and paying for) home care or seeking inpatient care at the VA or other institutions. Although 80% of veterans aged 55 and over have group or private health insurance and 90% aged 65 and over have Medicare coverage (U.S. Veterans Administration, 1984), these insurance systems provide little if any coverage for long-term care, either in the patient's home or in long-term-care facilities. Without the VA system of care, veterans and their families, like other families, face the necessity of spending their financial resources on long-term care until they reach "medical indigence." At that point they may or may not be eligible for Medicaid, depending on their age and the state where they live. Approximately 6% of male veterans aged 55 and over are covered by Medicaid, with the percentage rising from 2% at age 55 to 17% for those 75 and older. Thus there is a strong financial incentive for veterans and their families to turn to the VA for help and determination of eligibility for care.

Advocacy groups have called on the federal government to take steps to relieve the financial burden imposed by Alzheimer's disease and related disorders and to increase funding for research on causes and possible specific treatment. The fact that veterans as a class have access to VA care has led to efforts in Congress to extend special eligibility status to veterans with dementia. Such bills have been counter to the current eligibility structure in existing law; the proposed eligibility criteria in new legislation would have based care on a diagnostic category—i.e., dementia—rather than on service connection or financial status. Such a change in eligibility criteria could potentially overload the VA's inpatient capacity. With this criterion, the expanding number of potential patients, suggested by the demographics of dementia, could not all be admitted to present facilities for long-term care.

EDUCATION, RESEARCH AND
PATIENT-ENHANCEMENT ACTIVITIES

The VA is currently relying on improved organization of clinical, educational, and research resources to meet the growing challenges of dementia. The VA's approach has been to improve geriatric and gerontological staff skills across the entire spectrum of conditions requiring care, including dementia.

Geriatric Research, Education, and Clinical Centers (GRECCs)

Starting in 1974, the VA established Geriatric Research, Education and Clinical Centers (GRECCs) in VA medical centers across the nation. There are now 10 programs, located in Boston, Massachusetts; Durham, North Carolina; Gainesville, Florida; Little Rock, Arkansas; Minneapolis, Minnesota; St. Louis, Missouri; Seattle, Washington; and Palo Alto, Sepulveda, and West Los Angeles, California. The GRECC programs focus attention on the "geriatric imperative" generated by the aging of America's veterans by increasing knowledge of the aging process, by improving the quality of care for elderly veterans, and by attracting creative investigators, educators, and clinicians to careers in geriatrics and gerontology.

In FY 1985, funding for geriatric/gerontologic research by GRECC and affiliated VA staff grew by 23% from $11.6 million to $14.3 million, and research publications totaled 665. While most of this work was in biomedical areas, the proportion of health services research was 13% of the total number of publications.

Directions of Research

Dementia was the research target in more than 70 VA projects in FY 1985. Some titles illustrate the directions of investigations: "Neurological Aspects of Visual Tracking in Dementia"; "Sleep, Waking and EEG Patterns in Dementia"; "Biochemical Abnormalities in Cerebrospinal Fluid of Alzheimer Patients"; "HLA Genotypes in Alzheimer's Disease"; "Cholinergic Treatment of Memory Deficits in Dementia"; "A Family Study of Senile Dementia"; "Leukocyte Philothermal Response in Dementia of the Alzheimer Type"; "Psychological Characteristics of Presenile and Senile Dementia"; "Structured vs. Process Support Groups for Families of the Cognitively Impaired." Keeping in line with national research trends, the VA researchers are approaching the disease from multiple aspects.

Training

Professional training and education is another major activity of the GRECC program and the VA's Office of Academic Affairs. The VA sponsored 54 Geriatric Physician Fellowships in FY 1986. Of those, 28 fellows were in their first or second year of the two-year fellowship training programs at nine VA medical centers hosting GRECCs. A total of 128 have completed this fellowship program since its inception in 1978. Three GRECCs participated in training 116 health care professionals from a variety of disciplines in the Interdisciplinary Team Training in Geriatrics program. A total of 4,000 VA staff members took part in GRECC Enhancement continuing education the same year. In addition, many VA staff at other medical centers and non-VA community professionals participated in GRECC educational programs. The VA's Office of Academic Affairs also instituted a VA Gerontologic Nurse Fellowship program effective October 1, 1985. The two-year fellowship for graduating nursing students enrolled in doctoral-level programs was designed to produce expert geriatric nurse practitioners, educators, administrators, and researchers for leadership positions in long-term care for aging veterans. This doctoral-level program is an addition to the master's level clinical nurse specialist training program, now in its sixth year. In FY 1986, funding was provided for 118 master's level clinical nurse specialist student positions, including 68 in mental health and 43 in geriatrics. Subjects of educational programs mounted by GRECCs have included: clinical care of the elderly veteran with dementia; continuity of care for the aging veteran; drug monitoring in the elderly; techniques for the management of Alzheimer's disease; Alzheimer's disease: a conference of assessment and treatment of patients and caregivers; dementia and depression in the elderly; and current topics in geriatric neurology and psychiatry. A broad perspective of disciplines is represented in these educational programs.

Geriatric Evaluation Units

Another clinical resource in the VA's geriatrics program is the geriatric evaluation unit (GEU) (Rubenstein et al., 1984). GEUs are in operation at 71 VA medical centers, with more in the planning phases. GEUs provide comprehensive assessment of older patients who have multiple medical, functional, social, and psychological problems (Cheah & Beard, 1980). These assessments are performed by an interdisciplinary team consisting of at least a physician, a nurse, and a social worker. Patients with suspected dementia need careful evaluation before a definitive diagnosis of dementia can be made. This is necessary to rule out conditions such as delirium or depression and also to identify or rule out underlying conditions such as infection, metabolic deficiency, and tumors, for which there may be effective treatments (Council on Scientific Affairs, 1986). Patients with well-diagnosed dementing disease also require careful evaluation for concurrent illness and for nursing, psychological, and social needs (see also Winograd, Chapter 1; Burnside, Chapter 2; Brody, Chapter 6). Interdisciplinary teamwork is also needed to evaluate family and caregiver strengths and weaknesses and to work with families in making decisions about placement (see also Tune et al., Chapter 7). The GEU's comprehensive and interdisciplinary approach is an important resource for these purposes.

Dementia Units

Six VA medical centers have established patient-care units specifically for dementia patients. The units range in size from 16 to 44 beds and are usually located in the intermediate care sections of hospitals. They have designated areas where patients can pace or wander without disturbing others. At one such unit, transferring demented patients from a large ward to a cluster of single rooms reduced agitated behavior. However, the issue of whether demented patients are best placed in segregated, specialized units or in more general-purpose units with other patients is still unsettled clinically.

Dementia Education Projects and Publications

In response to the projected clinical needs associated with dementia, the Office of Geriatrics and Extended Care in the VA central office has undertaken or participated in significant educational projects to sensitize professionals, promulgate up-to-date information, and make the management of dementia more uniform and effective throughout the VA system.

The VA participated in the U.S. Department of Health and Human Services Task Force on Alzheimer's Disease, which produced the Report of the Secretary's Task Force on Alzheimer's Disease (U.S. Department of

Health and Human Services, 1984a). The report, an excellent summary of present knowledge and needs in research, training, and education, has been distributed to all VA medical centers.

VA staff members contributed expertise to the American Medical Association's panel on dementia. The end product was a clearly written consensus document for a general professional readership providing guidelines for diagnosis and treatment of patients and dementia. The report was made available in June 1985 by the AMA's Council on Scientific Affairs and published in 1986 (American Medical Association, 1986).

VA staff also took part in the deliberations of an interagency working group that produced a consensus paper on the clinical diagnosis of Alzheimer's disease (McKhann et al., 1984). VA staff prepared the section on distinctions between normal and pathological age differences in memory that is widely used in clinical training as well as by researchers (Fozard, 1985).

In addition to these activities, a series of internal seminars and workgroup conferences on dementia were held under VA auspices in collaboration with the Kellogg International Scholarship Program of the University of Michigan's Institute on Gerontology. VA and European experts prepared a set of "Recommendations [to the VA] for Patient Care, Research and Training," which were published and distributed to all VA medical centers (University of Michigan, 1985). Also distributed was a special issue of the *Danish Medical Bulletin* containing papers on Alzheimer's disease presented at the U.S. seminars and at a World Health Organization conference in Denmark (Danish Medical Association, 1985). In response to the "Recommendations," the VA has, in collaboration with several medical schools, established a brain bank to study brain tissue of dementia victims after death. The VA has also launched studies on the diagnosis of dementia and neurochemical patterns, comparisons between early and late onset dementia, and the efficacy of patterns of care and support for patients and families.

Many of the issues raised by the VA for improving the diagnosis and treatment of veterans with dementia have been addressed in the VA information bulletin *Dementia: Guidelines for Diagnosis and Treatment* (U.S. Veterans Administration, 1985). The publication reflects the knowledge and views of more than 60 professionals in the form of written contributions, participation in consensus workgroups, or concurrence review. It is intended that the publication contribute significantly to the sensitization of VA staff members to issues surrounding dementia, including needs of patients and families, support groups, and ties between the VA and the community.

CONCLUSION

In recognition of the increasing prevalence of dementing illnesses, the Veterans Administration will continue to rely on research, staff education, and high-quality clinical care to address the pressing issues surrounding dementia. At the same time, continued collaboration and participation with other federal agencies, universities, private organizations, and community groups will be essential in order to ensure that quality medical care is provided on a timely basis to eligible veterans.

Acknowledgments: Jacqueline Holmes and Adriana Masi for their secretarial support, and all of the members of the VA staff who contributed to this article and who have cared for patients with Alzheimer's disease.

11
The Role of Human Services

Janet S. Sainer

The search for answers to the mysteries surrounding Alzheimer's disease engages professionals from a wide spectrum of disciplines in science and health. What of social services? What role can they play?

While the all-important quest to define and understand Alzheimer's disease goes on, there is a unique and critical function that can be performed by community human service agencies: providing support and assistance to the families who must cope daily with the burdens imposed by the disease (see also Brody, Chapter 6; Tune et al., Chapter 7; Reveley, Chapter 8). This is an important area of knowledge that needs to be expanded.

Alzheimer's disease, without doubt, deals a crushing blow to the mind, body, and spirit of its victims—some 1 to 2 million of them across the nation (U.S. Department of Health and Human Services, 1984b).

But just as it ravages the patient, Alzheimer's disease also takes its toll on the patient's family. Most family members continue to care for their relatives at home for many years after a medical diagnosis has been made. In that time span, the family experiences progressively demanding needs: information about the disease; advice and direction on financial and legal matters; individual counseling; respite care; in-home services; help relating to public benefits and entitlements; and assistance in institutional placement. The needs are as endless as the evolving problems the Alzheimer patient presents in his or her downward course of impairment.

As one middle-aged daughter who is caring for her father has related: "I would urge each and every family member close to the victim to seek help. My father may continue to live within the shell of his body for years or he may die next week, but the well members of the family must learn to cope, not only with the disease, but with the real world we all live in."

The family becomes caught up in the dilemma of increasing demands and decreasing resources. The single most agonizing question becomes: Where can we go for help?

Until quite recently the community's understanding of Alzheimer's disease was very limited, and there was little public awareness of the devastating impact of this disease.

Families, overwhelmed and overburdened by care demands and stigmatized by a misunderstood degenerative disease process, tended to close themselves off and to cope silently, reluctant to seek assistance and unaware of what help was available. Similarly, professionals frequently have been unaware of resources offered by various health and human service agencies outside their own discipline or agency that can be helpful to Alzheimer families.

A RESPONSE BY A MUNICIPALITY

This chapter describes one locality's response to the fact that today Alzheimer's disease and related disorders present issues that can no longer be ignored by any field. Recognizing this, the City of New York held its first Mayoral Conference on Alzheimer's Disease and Related Disorders in 1983 under the auspices of the New York City Department for the Aging.

The Department for the Aging serves 1.3 million older adults (60 and older) and has been extensively engaged in issues of long-term care. Among these elderly, we estimate that there are 50,000 Alzheimer patients living in the community, with an additional 20,000 in institutions. At the time the Department for the Aging was preparing for its first city-sponsored conference, it had limited direct experience with Alzheimer patients and families. Yet as the federally designated Area Agency on Aging and also the municipal agency charged with coordinating services for the aging in New York City, the Department for the Aging was in a position to convene a group of experts from medical, health, social service, nursing home, aging, and academic arenas, as well as family caregivers and representatives of the Alzheimer's Disease and Related Disorders Association (ADRDA), to plan the first Mayoral Conference.

It soon became clear to the many organizations engaged in this effort that a resource directory of all agencies providing services for Alzheimer patients and families should be prepared and made ready for distribution at the conference. This undertaking led not only to the establishment of a centralized knowledge base of available services but also was the foundation of a citywide coalition concerned with Alzheimer patients and their families.

Moreover, as the development of the resource directory took on sharper focus, it highlighted the fact that not only were there gaps in the current service system, but that there was a need for a central mechanism to coordinate existing resources and to work toward developing new service initiatives to meet the needs of Alzheimer families.

It was appropriate that the Department for the Aging, an arm of the municipal government, be the central coordinating mechanism. Upon securing financial support from the Brookdale Foundation and the City of New York, the New York City Alzheimer's Resource Center was established in March 1984.

The Resource Center initially targeted its priorities toward informing families of its availability, linking them with existing community resources, and developing services that were not being provided by other organizations. Its activities were conducted in cooperation with the Greater New York chapter of ADRDA. The Center distributed informational material about Alzheimer's disease already available through ADRDA and referred clients with medical and clinical issues to the medical diagnostic centers in the city.

The Center built on its special capabilities as an Area Agency on Aging and social service resource, particularly in the areas of public benefits and entitlements and community-based services for the elderly.

SERVICES PROVIDED BY THE NEW YORK CITY ALZHEIMER'S RESOURCE CENTER

Today the Center is the only municipally sponsored agency of its kind in the nation and is engaged in three major areas of activity. First, it provides direct service for family members who need a range of supportive services, not the least of which is one-to-one counseling for caregivers. It offers information about and referral to medical diagnostic centers, family support groups, ADRDA activities, community social services, and adult daycare and respite programs. Guidance and intensive follow-up assistance are also given on obtaining public benefits, securing in-home services, and facilitating institutional placement.

Recognizing the complexity of legal and financial issues facing

Alzheimer families, the New York City Alzheimer's Resource Center recently initiated a legal-service program to assist family members who cannot otherwise afford private counsel for reimbursement issues, Medicaid eligibility, durable power of attorney, estate planning, and other legal matters.

The Resource Center's second major area of service is to the professional community. The Center offers technical assistance and guidance to the staff of medical and social service agencies, senior-center directors, clergy, physicians, and private-sector personnel directors, among others. It serves as a centralized information resource for those from various disciplines and provides linkage to other community services.

The third area of concentration for the New York City Alzheimer's Resource Center is its broad public education program. It relies extensively on the media to convey its message. The Center views its public education function as sensitizing the community at large to the problems and issues related to Alzheimer's disease as well as to the resources available in New York City.

The Center conducts workshops and seminars for community groups and for those who may be in contact with Alzheimer families but do not have the training or expertise to respond sufficiently to their needs. In addition, the Center has convened three large-scale Mayoral Conferences targeted primarily to family caregivers.

The Center has found that its recent publications are extremely useful for family members and professional providers. Its resource directory, *Alzheimer's Disease: Where To Go For Help In New York City* (New York City Department for the Aging, 1987), lists available and appropriate services and programs. *Caring: A Family Guide to Managing the Alzheimer's Patient at Home* (New York City Department for the Aging, 1985), is a 100-page illustrated guidebook that provides concrete, step-by-step suggestions for family caregivers on how to cope with the patient through various stages of the disease. Also available is *Agendas for Action: The Aging Network Responds to Alzheimer's Disease* (New York City Department for the Aging's Alzheimer's Resource Center and the Brookdale Foundation, 1986), a reference book describing the New York City Alzheimer's Resource Center and Alzheimer's programs and services provided by 244 State Offices and Area Agencies on Aging in 46 states across the nation.

The New York City Alzheimer's Resource Center is fortunate to have an outstanding advisory board composed of leaders of the city's medical community, aging network, academic gerontological centers, ADRDA leadership, the legal world, and nursing home administrators, as well as other health professionals and family caregivers. They serve in a planning and policy capacity as well as being speakers, workshop leaders, or consultants for the Center's major educational endeavors. Their organizations are important referral resources. They also engage in advocacy for legislation and research on behalf of Alzheimer families.

During its first 15 months of operation, the Center responded to more than 6,000 individuals; an additional 3,000 were reached through public education conferences and seminars.

Thirty percent of the Center's weekly requests were for general information and literature, 15% were for referrals to medical diagnostic centers, 28% were related to home care services, and 27% were in relation to nursing home placement.

Approximately 38% of all requests for assistance required multiple follow-up activities and intervention as well as supportive services from voluntary and public agencies. Being part of city government has enabled the Center to have access to other critical public systems—Medicaid, home care, hospitals, the City Department of Social Services, the Police Department, and the Department of Mental Health.

COLLABORATIVE EFFORTS ON BEHALF OF ALZHEIMER FAMILIES

As the Center has grown in capacity, expertise, and experience, it has continued to understand full well that achieving the goals of sound, solid coordination of resources, expansion of services, and effective advocacy cannot be accomplished alone. The success of these collaborative efforts is dependent upon the commitment and cooperation of the leadership of all social service agencies that have an impact on Alzheimer's disease.

But success hinges on more than community-based collaborative efforts of social service agencies. Other professional disciplines—medicine, health care, law, psychology, nursing—must also be involved if a community is to be a true resource to the victims of Alzheimer's disease and to their caregivers. Information sharing among disciplines is essential. Doctors and nurses caring for Alzheimer patients can be assisted by knowing about social, legal, and financial services that may benefit patients and their families. Similarly, as new knowledge about the disease becomes available, this information should be disseminated to social service agencies to help shape and guide their programs.

We must develop in every community a continuum of care, ranging from in-home services to institutional care and involving professionals in many fields. No single agency or individual has the capability to provide all that is necessary for the complex needs of Alzheimer patients and their families. We must, therefore, mesh multiple resources available in the community; advocate for expanded research activities and new diagnostic knowledge to solve the riddle of Alzheimer's disease; and work in the legislative arena on behalf of Alzheimer families to ensure that they do not become a pauperized generation, both financially and emotionally.

There is a clear cry for help from those whose lives are altered by this disease—and we must answer that cry now.

PART IV
Research

12

Research Issues and Neuropsychology

Asenath LaRue

An important but difficult aspect of research on treatments for Alzheimer's disease is the selection of instruments to measure changes in cognition and behavioral symptoms. The challenge is to identify quantitative tests that are valid, reliable, brief, comprehensible to patients with cognitive impairment, and sensitive to the small improvements that may result from currently available therapies. In principle, neuropsychological tests are well suited for measuring response to treatment in Alzheimer's disease, since they are designed specifically to assay cognitive functions affected by brain impairment. However, so few of these tests have been normed for aged samples that their psychometric properties in Alzheimer's disease investigations are largely a matter of conjecture. Perhaps because of this, a confusing array of outcome measures, including mental-status exams and behavioral rating scales as well as many different neuropsychological tests, are represented in the literature to date.

The aim of this chapter is to provide an introduction to some of the decisions that must be made in selecting neuropsychological tests for treatment investigations. The discussion is organized around a series of questions that underscore the link between test selection and the overall scientific framework of an investigation. An underlying assumption is that there are no general "best tests" for studying Alzheimer's disease; consequently, no attempt will be made to prescribe a specific treatment outcome battery. However, because most current interventions are aimed at improving memory, examples of different options for memory evaluation have been included.

Drugs are listed by both brand name and generic name in the Drug Index.

173

WHO WILL BE STUDIED?

By definition, all patients diagnosed with Alzheimer's disease have certain cognitive and behavioral deficits in common; for example, loss of general intellectual ability, memory impairment, and deficits in higher-order cognitive abilities such as language, visuospatial processing, and abstraction (DSM-III-R) (American Psychiatric Association, 1987; McKhann et al., 1984). Nonetheless, striking differences exist among demented individuals that need to be considered in choosing assessment batteries.

Severity of Illness

The most important determinant of individual differences is severity or stage of dementia. For patients who have reached moderate levels of illness, most traditional neuropsychological tests are simply too difficult to be validly administered (Hughes CP et al., 1982; Reisberg & Ferris, 1982). Although this is well known, many Alzheimer's disease treatment studies continue to include test batteries beyond the abilities of the patients being evaluated, with the result that a high proportion of subjects obtain zero scores on some or all of the measures.

Using neuropsychological tests that are too difficult jeopardizes treatment outcome research in a number of ways: (1) statistical power is lost; (2) the number and scope of behaviors that can be correlated with other study indices is restricted; and (3) chances are increased that uncontrolled factors might operate to produce a spurious treatment effect.

We recently encountered this problem in a study of the effects of a calcium channel blocker on cognitive functions in Alzheimer's disease and multiinfarct dementia. The test battery was selected by the corporation funding the research and consisted of six measures assessing motor, language, visuospatial, and memory skills. However, the screening criteria called for the inclusion of severely demented patients, that is, those with Mini-Mental State scores (Folstein et al., 1975) (see Appendix 1) as low as 4. We found that two of the cognitive tests were too difficult for nearly all of the patients, and the most severely impaired subjects obtained zero scores on all but one measure. The battery was time consuming and frequently frustrating for the patients, in addition to being psychometrically ill suited for detecting potential improvements.

In general, tests of intermediate difficulty are most likely to be sensitive to group and treatment differences (Chapman & Chapman, 1978), and outcome measures should be selected with this in mind.

Different tests may be needed for each new sample, or even for different individuals within the same sample. An example of this is provided in Table 12.1, where baseline memory-test data for 10 Alzheimer patients are summarized (Mohs et al., 1982). For some of the subjects, the word recognition test came closest to meeting the intermediate-difficulty criterion; that is, performance was above the chance level of 12 correct, but below a perfect score of 24. For other patients, picture recognition was the only measure to yield a score in the intermediate range. In light of this variability, Mohs and his colleagues (1982) recommended that the effectiveness of treatment be assessed on an individual-subject basis, using either word or picture recognition as the outcome measure.

The scores in Table 12.1 also illustrate how difficult verbal recall tests can be for Alzheimer patients: 70% had zero or near-zero scores when they attempted to recall a list of 10 words. Evaluation of recall can be very helpful diagnostically, since dementia patients' performance is usually clearly worse than that of healthy elderly people or depressed or anxious patients without organic mental disorder (Inglis, 1959; La Rue et al., 1986a; E. Miller, 1977; Storandt et al., 1984). In treatment studies, however, tests must be able to detect decline as well as improvement, and verbal recall tasks that yield very low scores initially should generally be excluded from test–retest batteries.

TABLE 12.1 Baseline Memory-Test Performance of 10 Patients with Clinically Diagnosed Alzheimer's Disease

Patient	10-word recall	24-word recognition	24-picture recognition
1	2.0	18.7	22.7
2	5.6	13.7	23.5
3	0.4	20.0	22.0
4	0.0	14.0	24.0
5	0.0	16.0	14.3
6	2.5	19.3	24.0
7	0.7	19.0	23.0
8	0.0	12.0	17.3
9	0.0	15.7	19.3
10	0.0	11.0	14.3
Mean	1.1	15.9	20.4

Note: Scores were averaged over one or more learning trials.

Source: "Defining Treatment Efficacy in Patients with Alzheimer's Disease," by R. C. Mohs, W. G. Rosen, and K. L. Davis. In S. Corkin, K. L. Davis, J. H. Growdon, E. Usdin, & R. J. Wurtman (eds.), *Alzheimer's Disease: A Report of Progress in Research*, Vol. 19: *Aging*. New York: Raven Press. © 1982. Used with permission.

Nonetheless, there are some published investigations in which tests of verbal learning and recall have been successfully used to measure treatment outcome. For example, Peters and Levin (1979) were able to demonstrate differential improvement in verbal recall when Alzheimer patients were given a combination of physostigmine and lecithin as opposed to taking either of these compounds alone. The outcome measure was a version of the Buschke–Fuld Selective Reminding Task (Buschke & Fuld, 1974), which requires the subject to try to memorize a short list of familiar nouns. Several recall trials are given, with the subject being reminded at the end of each trial of only those items that he or she had forgotten (i.e., "selective" reminding). This test is a sensitive measure of a patient's ability to transfer and store information in long-term or secondary memory, a process that appears to be one of the core areas of deficit in Alzheimer's disease (E. Miller, 1977; Wilson et al., 1983). Although the selective reminding task was very difficult for these patients, baseline testing showed that their performance improved with practice and that they were able to learn an average of 4 out of 12 words. It is also important to note that verbal intelligence was still fairly well preserved in this sample (Verbal IQ score range = 91–115).

The surest method for avoiding a mismatch between sample characteristics and test requirements is to pilot the test battery with patients similar to those you hope to treat. An alternative is to try to replicate procedures of related investigations, such as the study described above. This is only feasible, of course, if the prior study provided detailed descriptions of subject-selection criteria, so that new subjects with the same global dementia severity can be obtained.

If only moderately to severely impaired patients are available for study, most traditional neuropsychological tests should be excluded as outcome measures, substituting, instead, simple mental-status questionnaires (e.g., the Mini-Mental State Examination [Folstein et al., 1975]) (see Appendix 1), observer-rated cognitive or behavior scales (e.g., the Brief Cognitive Rating Scale [Reisberg et al., 1983c], the Alzheimer's Disease Assessment Scale [Mohs et al., 1983], the Sandoz Clinical Assessment–Geriatric [SCAG] [Venn, 1983], Inventory of Psychic and Somatic Complaints–Elderly [Raskin & Rae, 1981]), or, possibly, simple tasks adapted from studies of nonhuman primates, as recommended by Albert and Moss (1984).

Disease Progression

In intervention studies with long-term follow-ups, changes in severity of illness over time can further compromise the validity of neuropsychological testing procedures. As symptoms progress, tests that were initially appropriate become more difficult and may no longer be capable of detecting a group difference of the same magnitude as that initially observed. An investigator could easily conclude that a beneficial effect of treatment was lost over time, when, in fact, it may simply be that the sensitivity of the measurement instrument has diminished.

Most Alzheimer treatment studies have focused on short-term outcomes, but evaluation of long-term effects will probably be a goal of the research on continuous intracranial cholinergic drug infusion (Harbaugh et al., 1984) and other chronic interventions that may be developed in the future.

A partial solution to the problem of changing test sensitivity would be to substitute simpler forms of the same type of test as the dementia worsens; for example, shortening the list of words in verbal recall tests or substituting recognition of pictures for recognition of words (Mohs, 1983). Absolute levels of performance could not be compared across test occasions, but treated and untreated groups could be validly contrasted at each point in time.

Patterns of Cognitive Deficit

Individual differences in patterns of cognitive deficit also have implications for test selection. Deficits in learning and memory are still considered to be the earliest and most striking problem for most individuals with Alzheimer's disease, but some patients have significant language impairment as an early sign, whereas others have disproportionate deficits in visuospatial abilities (Albert & Moss, 1984; Kirschner et al., 1984; Naugle et al., 1985). If subjects with each of these different symptom patterns are included in a study, variability in neuropsychological test scores will be increased, particularly if the sample size is small.

Deficits in higher-order cognitive functions such as language or visuospatial perception can indirectly bias performance on tests of learning and memory that frequently serve as key outcome measures in Alzheimer treatment investigations (Albert & Moss, 1984). For example, in another recent drug study in our laboratory, four of the five tests of memory required a verbal response (listing words, labeling pictures, recalling names, and repeating numbers). For a few of the subjects, poor performance appeared to be due as much to word-finding problems as to memory loss per se. Another individual with Parkinson-like symptoms responded extremely slowly, and our estimate of his memory abilities might well have been colored by this psychomotor retardation.

It is too early to know if there are distinct subtypes of Alzheimer's disease or if variations in cognitive test patterns can be used to identify subtypes (Jorm, 1985). At present, screening for subjects in treatment investigations should be conducted carefully, with the aim of minimizing individual differences in patterns of cognitive deficit. This can be accomplished in a rough manner through the use of an instrument such as the Mini-Mental State Examination (Folstein et al., 1975). In addition to establishing cutoffs based on total score (e.g., 18–23 correct out of a possible total of 30), performance on different sections of the test should be examined to screen for patterns of deficit. Many early Alzheimer patients will miss only attention/calculation and delayed recall questions, and, perhaps, some orientation items. Others, however, will miss some of the written language items or be unable to copy the two-dimensional design, in addition to having problems with memory. These patients are likely to obtain disproportionately low scores on verbal and nonverbal neuropsychological tests, respectively, and their inclusion in a small study sample might complicate detection of treatment-related change.

Specific Psychiatric Complications

Coexisting psychiatric symptoms can also be an important source of variability in neuropsychological test performance. There have not been any large-scale investigations addressing the prevalence of these symptoms in adequately diagnosed Alzheimer patients, but smaller clinical studies have reported that 30% to 50% of these patients have symptoms of depression, 20% to 80% are agitated, at least on occasion, and 20% to 30% exhibit psychotic symptoms (Coblentz et al., 1973; Mohs et al., 1982; Sim & Sussman, 1962) (see also Winograd, Chapter 1; Satlin & Cole, Chapter 3; Cohen, Chapter 5).

Each of the psychiatric problems noted above has been linked to cognitive impairments in older patients *without* dementia (Caine, 1981; Kiloh, 1961; Weingartner & Silberman, 1982; Wells, 1979). We found that more than 20% of a sample of depressed elderly inpatients who were not demented obtained very low scores (i.e., <20) on the Mini-Mental State (La Rue et al., 1986b) (see Appendix 1); none was able to recall three objects after a brief delay, most missed some basic orientation questions, and 75% could not accurately copy a two-dimensional design. These cognitively impaired patients were more likely to be delusional, highly anxious, or agitated than other, equally depressed subjects who did not have cognitive problems.

If agitation or psychotic features can diminish cognitive performance to this extent in patients without dementia, it stands to reason that they could also affect cognition among Alzheimer patients. In treatment studies, therefore, screening procedures should identify the extent of psychiatric symptoms as well as cognitive deficits. The Hamilton Depression Scale (Hamilton, 1960) (see Appendix 7) has been used to screen for depression in mild-to-moderately impaired Alzheimer patients. This is an observer-rated instrument assessing dysphoric mood, loss of interest in activities, and vegetative signs of depression; it also includes items measuring agitation and anxiety. Another potentially useful instrument in the Global Assessment of Psychiatric Symptoms–Elderly (GAPS–E). This 19-item scale taps a wide range of psychiatric features, including depressed mood, anxiety and agitation, and psychotic symptoms; it has been included in studies with geriatric patients with clinical diagnoses of dementia or depression (Raskin & Rae, 1981).

Because dementia interferes with patients' ability to evaluate their condition and to communicate their feelings to others, the scores obtained with these psychiatric rating scales must be considered rough estimates. Nonetheless, including such scales provides the investigator with a shorthand notation for describing the extent of coexisting psychiatric symptoms in a study sample. In addition, there may be treatments that enhance cognition by reducing anxiety or psychosis, and quantitative scales are needed to evaluate this possibility.

Premorbid Abilities and Demographic Characteristics

Among normal aging people, differences in education, occupation, and overall intellectual level can strongly affect performance on neuropsychological tests. Sex and age differences are also commonly observed. Effects of these factors are still likely to be observed among patients in the early phases of Alzheimer's disease, even though progressive brain impairment eventually obscures individual differences.

Educational level has been shown to influence scores on mental-status screening examinations such as the Kahn–Goldfarb Mental Status Questionnaire (Gurland, 1981), the Short Portable Mental Status Questionnaire (Pfeiffer, 1975), and the Mini-Mental State Examination (Anthony et al., 1982). On the Mini-Mental State, a high proportion of subjects without dementia, but with an eighth-grade education or less, obtained total scores below 23, the typical cutoff used in screening for dementia or delirium (Anthony et al., 1982). The same was true for black as opposed to white subjects, and for elderly as opposed to middle-aged patients (Anthony et al., 1982). Clinically, we have observed that many well-educated patients with professional occupational backgrounds score above the cutoff of 23, even though Alzheimer's disease is suggested by a history of gradual functional decline and poor performance on other, more sensitive tests.

On neuropsychological tests, background factors may account for some of the variations in the Alzheimer test profiles discussed above. Naugle and colleagues (1985) found that some clinically diagnosed Alzheimer patients had relatively well-preserved verbal skills and others, fairly intact nonverbal skills; the average level of education was higher in both of these groups than for patients whose test performance was more globally impaired. Sex differences were also observed, with more women falling into the verbally intact subgroup and more men obtaining a visuospatially intact profile.

The practical implication of these findings is that background factors, so important in studies of normal aging, must also be considered in screening for Alzheimer's disease treatment investigations. Cutoff scores on standardized mental-status exams should be adjusted upward if you are planning to study well-educated or premorbidly superior subjects, and downward if the reverse is true. Similarly, it is important to recognize that many published studies have focused on Alzheimer patients who were initially very bright (Weingartner et al., 1981); the neuropsychological tests included in these studies may prove too difficult for less able subjects, even if the two groups could be matched for overall levels of dementia.

Summary

The importance of various sampling issues for selection of test instruments cannot be overemphasized. If treatments are to be evaluated by comparing outcomes for different groups, then a good strategy is to screen subjects carefully so that they will be similar to each other on all variables other than the treatment per se (e.g., level of dementia, concomitant psychiatric symptoms, education). Whether group or individual analyses are performed, it is advisable to pilot test memory tasks and other neuropsychological measures to be certain that baseline scores are in the intermediate range, allowing for both improvements or declines as a result of intervention.

WHAT WILL THE TREATMENT BE?

Alzheimer's disease affects almost all aspects of cognition and behavior, but existing treatments are typically limited as to the range of behaviors they might reasonably be expected to improve. The more that is known or hypothesized in advance about the mode of action of a given intervention, the more closely the assessment battery can be tailored to detect the outcome (Weingartner, 1985).

Cholinergic Agents

The most systematic research to date on experimental treatments for Alzheimer's disease has examined effects of cholinergic precursors, agonists, and antagonists. The early literature has been summarized by Barbeau and colleagues (1979) and Bartus and colleagues (1982), and new studies in this area appear to be continuing at a steady rate (Harbaugh et al., 1984; Johns et al., 1985).

Neuropsychological tests have been used as outcome measures in most studies of cholinergic agents. Two approaches have been taken to the selection of test batteries: (1) a focused approach, using one or more measures of learning and memory (Mohs & Davis, 1982; Peters & Levin, 1979); and (2) a comprehensive approach, assessing attention, language, or visuospatial functions in addition to learning and memory (Ferris et al., 1979).

Focused batteries have several general advantages, not the least of which is brevity of administration. If only one or two measures are used, selection can be limited to instruments of known reliability, validity, and sensitivity; it is also easier to develop alternate forms of the battery. The only major disadvantage to this approach is that a true treatment effect might go unnoticed (Type II error) if the battery does not include an index of the affected ability or behavior.

Comprehensive batteries reduce the odds that an unanticipated treatment effect will be overlooked. In addition, a treatment study with a negative outcome is more convincing if a comprehensive assessment battery was used. If many tests are given, however, there is likely to be redundancy among the measures that needlessly increases administration time. Also, the odds of finding at least one significant outcome are increased, even though this may be due only to chance (Type I error).

Regarding cholinergic agonists and antagonists, studies with animals and healthy young adults suggest that manipulation of the central cholinergic system has fairly direct effects on learning and memory, especially on long-term storage of new information. Other aspects of cognition (e.g., attention, short-term memory, visuospatial perception, etc.) do not appear to be directly affected. Therefore, in cholinergic treatment studies, brief batteries assessing learning and memory are empirically defensible as well as efficient. Investigations with many tests have not added substantially to knowledge in this area, although they have helped to cement the impression that some agents (especially precursors such as choline or lecithin) are ineffective in treating Alzheimer symptoms (Ferris et al., 1979).

As Weingartner (1985) indicates, studies of the effects of catecholaminergic agents on cognition might require different outcome measures than cholinergic investigations. Catecholaminergic agents affect arousal, which, in turn, can influence memory performance. The assessment approach that Weingartner (1985) recommends includes evaluation of noncognitive factors (e.g., arousal or mood) as well as selected cognitive functions in order to examine both direct and indirect effects of different chemical treatments.

Other Interventions

Most of the treatment studies with Alzheimer patients have not had a clearly articulated rationale, and the varied assessment batteries represented in this research seem to reflect this scientific ambiguity.

For example, there have been many nonsomatic treatments advocated for Alzheimer symptoms, including individual and group psychotherapy, reality orientation, exercise therapy, and cognitive-skills training. However, neither the subject characteristics nor outcome measures have been adequately described in the literature on these interventions (Eisdorfer et al., 1981; Liston & Jarvik, in press; Zarit & Anthony, 1986).

One of the few investigations of this type to use a neuropsychological outcome measure was conducted by Diesfeldt and Diesfeldt-Groenendijk (1977). The study was undertaken to investigate the clinical impression that psychogeriatric patients seemed more cheerful and alert after they had taken part in physical exercises. Performance on a verbal free recall test was measured before and after physical exercise in a sample of 40 nursing home residents with organic brain syndrome, and a significant improvement in test scores was observed.

In a more recent investigation, Brinkman and colleagues (1982) studied the effects of a combined course of memory-training exercises and lecithin supplementation in 10 clinically diagnosed Alzheimer patients. They failed to find sustained improvement on the Buschke–Fuld Selective Reminding Test (Buschke & Fuld, 1974) as a result of this intervention.

Both of these studies leave a number of questions unanswered. In the Diesfeldt and Diesfeldt-Groenendijk (1977) investigation, it is not clear why a learning and memory test was chosen to measure the effects of exercise when the clinical observations prompting the study pertained to changes in mood and arousal. In the second study, the memory-training procedures were only sketchily described and the rationale for expecting improvement with training was not sufficiently developed. Subjects may have been incapable of learning the memory strategies, since this type of mnemonic requires abstraction and reasoning ability. Alternatively, they may have understood the mnemonics initially but failed to apply them when tested on the selective reminding task.

Problems with theoretical and procedural clarity are by no means limited to the literature on psychosocial interventions. Many drug treatment studies with Alzheimer patients have also had vague rationales or inadequate procedures (e.g., see Hughes et al., 1976, for a critique of studies of dihydroergotoxine). Under these circumstances, it is difficult to explain conflicting outcomes or to plan a further investigation to resolve ambiguities.

Summary

Given our rudimentary knowledge of the pathophysiology of Alzheimer's disease, some guesswork is bound to be involved in research on symptomatic treatments. Ideally, however, test selection should be dictated by a model of brain–behavior relations that encompasses the treatment of interest. At this point in time, a series of small-scale, theoretically focused investigations, as in the research on cholinergic agents, would be preferable to broadly construed studies of clinicians' best hunches.

WHEN, WHERE, AND HOW ARE THE PATIENTS TO BE EVALUATED?

Before assessment instruments can be selected, it is also important to know how many test sessions are anticipated and how closely spaced consecutive sessions will be.

There are two types of potential practice effects that need to be taken into account. The first occurs when a subject recalls or recognizes an item that has been previously administered and either remembers the answer or requires less time or effort to figure it out. The second type, called "reactivity" (Schaie, 1983), involves a more global change in a subject's behavior as a result of having been previously tested. For example, a person may be more relaxed during a second or third test session simply because the procedures and examiner are more familiar.

In general, the more frequent and closely spaced the evaluations, the more serious is the possibility of significant practice effects. Testing done to evaluate short-acting medications (e.g., intravenous physostigmine) or to correlate with expensive, time-limited assessments (e.g., positron emission tomography) are two examples of situations where several closely spaced assessments are likely to be needed. Alternate forms should be used for all tests if the battery is administered once a day or more. This precludes the use of many neuropsychological tests (e.g., the Wechsler Adult Intelligence Scale [Wechsler, 1955, 1981] or measures from the

Halstead–Reitan battery [Reitan & Davison, 1974]). It is also a question-able practice to use measures with a single alternate form (e.g., the Wechsler Memory Scale [Wechsler, 1945]) if there are several closely spaced reevaluations.

To reduce the possibility of obtaining test–retest changes due to nonspecific factors, it is helpful to schedule several baseline assessments using different forms of the target test battery. This allows subjects to become familiar with the general procedure and can reduce variability in scores. With a more stable baseline, treatment-related changes might be more easily detected.

The setting in which testing takes place can also influence the choice of test instruments. Computerized assessment procedures have been rec-ommended as particularly useful for evaluating drug efficacy in dementia (Branconnier et al., 1981b), but this approach might not be feasible if patients need to be seen in their homes or long-term-care facilities. In addition, in studies involving long-term evaluation of treatment out-comes, it may be necessary to change the site of evaluation over time. In this situation as well, any assessment requiring extensive instrumentation would be impractical.

The question of how the testing is to be accomplished raises several practical considerations, any of which could influence the reliability of outcomes. One of the most important of these "nuts-and-bolts" issues concerns duration of test sessions. With lengthy batteries, subjects usual-ly require several breaks to minimize fatigue. We generally limit neuro-psychological testing to an hour per day for cognitively impaired patients, with one break in the middle of the session. Some patients, however, can only concentrate for 10 or 15 minutes at a time, and others will only consent to participate if all of the testing can be completed in one day. These variations probably influence scores and increase the error variance.

Similarly, although most neuropsychological measures have stan-dardized instructions and administration procedures, patients with significant cognitive impairment are frequently "unstandard" in their ability to comprehend these procedures. Examiners respond to this with varying degrees of informal prompting and clarification. We have found that subjects obtain higher scores on the average when tested by some of our examiners as opposed to others, in spite of the fact that all of our staff have substantial training and experience in working with elderly patients. To keep this variation to a minimum, additional training can be helpful, advising examiners of the different exceptions to standard pro-cedures that are likely to arise and agreeing in advance on methods for handling these situations.

SUMMARY AND CONCLUSIONS

It is clear that there is no single solution to the problem of selecting a neuropsychological test battery to evaluate a treatment outcome. However, different options can be prioritized if adequate information is available on the characteristics of the sample to be studied, the predicted scope of the treatment effect, and the timing and logistics of the assessment situation.

The studies for which it is easiest to select a test battery are the ones that have clear scientific rationales. If an investigator has well-delineated hypotheses about how a treatment works, then tests can generally be found to measure the predicted outcomes.

To increase the probability of being able to detect small effects, care must be taken to minimize other sources of variability. Screening procedures are very important in this regard, as discussed above. Pilot testing to insure the absence of ceiling or floor effects may be needed, and multiple baseline assessments are desirable, although both may be costly to arrange if the study is being conducted with outpatients.

The extra work entailed in obtaining the right battery must be balanced against the personal and scientific costs of conducting a study that is methodologically inadequate. Patients are generally asked to attempt many difficult and frustrating tasks in conjunction with treatment research, and family members often need to take time away from work to accompany them. Neither can be justified if the study has little chance of contributing to our knowledge, which might well be the case if the wrong outcome measures are selected.

Grant support from: NIMH (Research Grant MH36205) and the Veterans Administration. The opinions expressed are not necessarily those of the Veterans Administration.

Acknowledgments: The assistance of Clara Neves and Anna Waldbaum in preparation of this chapter is greatly appreciated.

13
The Future: Some Speculations

Lissy F. Jarvik

WHERE RESEARCH HAS BROUGHT US

It is hazardous to speculate about future treatments of an illness as complex as Alzheimer's disease for which diagnostic criteria are in dispute, causes unknown, course variable, and even modifying influences entirely within the realm of conjecture. Since numerous reviews are available (Terry & Davies, 1980; Crook & Gershon, 1981; Reisberg, 1983; Wurtman, 1985a; Matsuyama et al., 1985; Roth & Iverson, 1986; Katzman, 1986), I will only highlight where research has brought us to date.

Age at Onset

The early literature tended to differentiate between presenile and senile forms of the disease on the basis of age at onset (i.e., before or after age 65). While the trend has been toward discarding the age distinction, evidence from a number of sources suggests the possibility of its reestablishment (Bondareff et al., 1982; Heston, 1983; Mountjoy et al., 1983).

Neurochemical Changes

The most consistent neurochemical finding has been a deficit in the enzyme choline acetyltransferase (CAT), which catalyzes the production of acetylcholine. Most of the cells making this chemical (cholinergic

Drugs are listed by both brand name and generic name in the Drug Index.

neurons in the nucleus basalis of Meynert) are seen to have been lost when the brains of Alzheimer patients are examined at autopsy. However, such loss occurs in other dementing illnesses as well (Rogers et al., 1985; Candy et al., 1983; Wisniewski et al., 1979).

Moreover, cells are also lost in other parts of the brain, that is, those needed for the highest level of intellectual functioning (association cortex), those concerned with the sense of smell (entorhinal cortex), and those intimately related to memory (hippocampus and limbic system). In the brains of Alzheimer patients who die at relatively young ages (in their sixties or even younger), most of the nerve cells providing the neurotransmitter noradrenalin to the cortex are no longer present in the locus ceruleus. Other brain substances have also been reported abnormal (notably somatostatin, serotonin, corticotropin releasing factor, nerve growth factor, and certain forms of ribonucleic acid [RNA]).

Infectious Agents

No infectious agent or virus has been identified—and it is not for lack of searching. In another form of dementia, Creutzfeldt-Jakob disease, the evidence is in favor of an unconventional slow virus infection despite the fact that this disease has a significant genetic component. Indeed, the same virus has also been identified in some patients with Gerstmann-Sträussler syndrome, a familial form of dementia with cerebellar ataxia. Unfortunately for research—fortunately for society—Creutzfeldt-Jakob disease is extremely rare, with an estimated yearly incidence of about one case per million (Masters et al., 1979; Brown, 1980). Animal studies with the scrapie agent (which, like the Creutzfeldt-Jakob disease agent, is classified as an "unconventional virus") showed that genetic factors, both in the animal and in the virus, control the development of brain changes. Indeed, different combinations of scrapie agent and mouse strain have different "signatures," which are only now beginning to be decoded (Carp et al., 1984).

Investigations of the Creutzfeldt-Jakob disease agent lag far behind those of scrapie. In one carefully studied five-generation pedigree (Rosenthal et al., 1976) with several autopsy-confirmed diagnoses of Creutzfeldt-Jakob disease, the findings were in accord with an autosomal dominant mode of transmission, that is, directly from parent to child with an average risk of 50% for children. A preexisting, genetically determined susceptibility may allow the virus to invade the body and the brain. Another possibility is that the virus is incorporated into the genetic material of the animal or person and transmitted from one generation to another until it is activated. Obviously, much work remains to be done before we will understand the genetics of Creutzfeldt-Jakob disease—and we know more about Creutzfeldt-Jakob disease than we do about Alzheimer's disease. Alzheimer's disease shares a number of pathological and clinical features with Creutzfeldt-Jakob disease and in some cases is also familial, exhibiting autosomal dominant inheritance. Further, there are some pedigrees containing both Alzheimer's disease and Creutzfeldt-Jakob disease; hence, we again have the possiblity of an infectious cause (Masters et al., 1981).

Immunology

Evidence suggesting immunological changes in Alzheimer's disease includes the following: immunoglobulins are found in the amyloid fibrils of the plaques; increased levels of brain reactive antibodies have been reported in the blood of patients with a clinical diagnosis of Alzheimer's disease; and, recently, a monoclonal antibody (ALZ-50) was found selective for Alzheimer's disease brain tissue relative to normal brain tissue (Wolozin et al., 1986). The antigen (A-68) has been demonstrated in the spinal fluid of Alzheimer patients and offers hope of a diagnostic test some years hence (Peter Davies, Albert Einstein College of Medicine, personal communication, 1986).

Abnormal Protein

In the amyloid plaque of Alzheimer's disease, an abnormal protein has been identified that closely resembles the protein of the paired helical filaments in the neurofibrillary tangles. Thus the hallmark lesions of Alzheimer's disease—plaques and tangles—share a common protein (Kidd et al., 1985). This protein seems to be different from the prion (proteinaceous infectious particle) identified in Creutzfeldt-Jakob disease and Gerstmann-Straüssler syndrome (Kitamoto et al., 1986). The composition of part of that protein is now being determined, especially the sequence of the 28 amino acids (Wong et al., 1985).

Gene Locus

Most recently, a gene coding for this amyloid protein and possibly an "Alzheimer gene" have been localized on chromosome 21 (Delabar et al., 1987; Goldgaber et al., 1987; Kang et al., 1987; Robakis et al., 1987; Selkoe et al., 1987; St. George-Hyslop et al., 1987; Tanzi et al., 1987). Chromosome 21 is present in three copies in Down's syndrome instead of the normal two, and Down's syndrome has long been associated with Alzheimer's disease. For example, most patients with Down's syndrome who live long enough develop the neuropathological changes characteristic of Alzheimer's disease (Jervis, 1948; Wisniewski et al., 1985), and an increased frequency of individuals with Down's syndrome is observed in Alzheimer's disease families. Localization to chromosome 21 of a gene which may have something to do with the cause of Alzheimer's disease fits in well with the observations described above and with the most recent research reports (M. Schweber, Boston University, personal communication, 1987).

Family Studies

Hereditary factors in Alzheimer's disease have been suspected for over half a century, and in a recent survey of the literature (Matsuyama et al., 1985), we found a total of 13 studies with information on familial risk. Combining data from these studies confirmed that first-degree relatives of individuals afflicted with Alzheimer's disease have about a threefold increase in the risk of developing the disease. Recently, Folstein and colleagues (Breitner & Folstein, 1984; Folstein et al., 1983) reported that language disorder and apraxia identify familial Alzheimer's disease, but this finding has not been replicated. Our own attempts to do so have been unsuccessful. The lone twin study (Kallmann, 1953) reported a concordance rate of 42.8% for identical and 8% for fraternal co-twins (i.e., in almost half the identical but less than 10% of the fraternal pairs, both twins had dementia). That finding supports a genetic component, but leaves room for substantial nongenetic influences.

In some families, the mode of inheritance is autosomal dominant (parent to child without skipping a generation); in others, it is not clear. In some families, an excess part of chromosome 21 (duplication) has been demonstrated (Delabar et al., 1987). And in yet others, it seems that a nonspecific predisposition to dementia may be inherited (Amaducci et al., 1986). Moreover, there are numerous patients without any affected relatives, even when the relatives survived long enough to manifest the disease (i.e., into their seventies and eighties). Granted the difficulty in getting accurate family histories, the occurrence of such "sporadic" cases is nonetheless well established, particularly for patients with late onset of the disease. Implications of the most recent genetic findings are discussed in the new international journal, *Alzheimer Disease and Associated Disorders* (A. J. Tobin, 1987).

Metals, Drugs, and Toxins

Much attention has been paid to *aluminum,* which has been found in high concentrations in the brains of patients with Alzheimer's disease and has been localized to the neurofibrillary tangle-bearing neurons and to the center of the plaques (Candy et al., 1986), the two major lesions of Alzheimer's disease. Currently, an attractive hypothesis is that a basic defect in mineral metabolism impairs the transport of neurofilament proteins and leads to the formation of neurofibrillary tangles. There may also be a relationship between aluminum and silicon dietary intake and plaque formation (Carlisle & Curran, 1987).

Clinical impression supports the association of *alcohol* in the development of Alzheimer's disease, but controlled data are lacking. Indeed, patients who have a history of significant alcohol use are generally excluded from research in Alzheimer's disease. Animal experiments indicate that alcohol may have selective actions on cholinergic and somatostatin systems (Mancillas et al., 1986). Juxtaposed with the ancient drug of alcohol, many of the modern potent *therapeutic drugs* have anticholinergic properties, as do the widely used *pesticides*. Contact with such anticholinergic compounds may aggravate the cholinergic deficit found in Alzheimer's disease.

Head Injury

Repeated head injury, such as that experienced by professional boxers, may lead to dementia pugilistica, a condition characterized by neuropathologic lesions similar to, but not identical with, those found in Alzheimer's disease (Corsellis, 1978). Specifically, there is an abundance of neurofibrillary tangles with few, if any, plaques; however, there is also septal fenestration, loss of pigment in substantia nigra with neurofibrillary tangles, and scarring of the cerebellar tonsils—none of which characterizes Alzheimer's disease. Reports vary on the frequency of a history of head trauma in patients with Alzheimer's disease, some failing to find a difference vis-à-vis controls, others finding an excess in patients (Heyman et al., 1983; Mortimer et al., 1985; Amaducci et al., 1986). Again, however, most studies of Alzheimer's disease exclude patients who have suffered head trauma.

WHERE RESEARCH MAY TAKE US

As illustrated by these highlights, scientists are investigating a variety of clues in their search for knowledge about Alzheimer's disease. And, unless serendipity intervenes, curing or preventing the disease will require a causally directed approach. Thus the first task is to try to identify possible causes from which rational treatments will emerge. The intense concentration of research on Alzheimer's disease has helped to focus us on that task; but, as the preceding pages show, we still have a long way to go before completing it. While awaiting definitive results, I will chance a few predictions; some are derived from available knowledge and fall into the category of informed guesses, others are more wildly speculative and, therefore, perhaps more intriguing.

First Prediction

We will come to view Alzheimer's disease as it is currently defined using DSM-III-R (American Psychiatric Association, 1987) criteria together with those of the NINCDS-ADRDA Work Group on the Diagnosis of Alzheimer's Disease (McKhann et al., 1984) *as the result of heterogeneous agents interacting with heterogeneous host factors.* Thus we will find that infectious agents, poisonous chemicals, nutritional deficiencies or excesses, head injury, anesthetics, and any number of other outside agents—now known or unknown—will produce Alzheimer's disease in individuals who have inherited or acquired a particular vulnerability, such as an abnormal gene for amyloid, a microtubular defect, or a suboptimal number of cholinergic neurons. Perhaps more than one exogenous factor may play a role in a given individual, for example, alcohol use, nutritional deficiency, and exposure to pesticide or heavy metals could easily occur in combination and participate in the pathogenesis of Alzheimer's disease. This prediction would help explain why it has been impossible thus far to disentangle the various interacting influences in the development of Alzheimer's disease. Our inability to make a definitive diagnosis of dementia of the Alzheimer type during the patient's lifetime remains a major handicap. The problem of antemortem diagnosis is currently being addressed by first-rate investigators, which leads to my second prediction.

Second Prediction

We will identify a series of biologic markers, specific for various subtypes of what we now call Alzheimer's disease. These markers will enable us to detect specific vulnerabilities; for example, one such marker, and one that has been of particular interest to our research group, may be a specific defect in one of the subcellular organelles, the *microtubular system.* Support for a *microtubular defect* in Alzheimer's disease includes the following. (1) An abnormality in microtubule organization may give rise to numerical chromosome aberrations. We found an increased frequency of such aberrations in patients with Alzheimer's disease, and so have others (Matsuyama et al., 1985; Whalley et al., 1982). (2) An abnormal microtubule immunofluorescent pattern has been reported in skin fibroblasts from a patient with Alzheimer's disease (Andia-Waltenbaugh & Puck, 1977). (3) A marked reduction (35%) in soluble tubulin, one component of microtubules, has been reported in the temporal cortex of five Alzheimer patients (Borthwick et al., 1985). (4) An intact mircotubule system is needed for directed cell migration (Malech et al., 1977), and a defect in temperature gradient directed cell migration has been observed in Alzheimer's disease (Jarvik et al., 1982). (5) Colchicine, a well-known microtubule disrupting agent, when added to cells obtained from cognitively intact individuals produced the abnormal temperature gradient directed cell migration response observed in Alzheimer's disease (Fu et al., 1986). (6) The major protein in paired helical filaments is the microtubule associated protein tau, which is known to enhance microtubular assembly (Grundke-Iqbal et al., 1986). (7) *In vitro* microtubule assembly was recently observed only in control and not in Alzheimer brains, most likely because of abnormal phosphorylation of the tau protein (Iqbal et al., 1986).

This second prediction implies that Alzheimer's disease will turn out to be a systemic disorder rather than a specific brain disease. I have held that point of view for some time (Jarvik, 1983), considering the brain a particularly sensitive rather than the sole target organ. The evidence in favor of cellular systems other than those of the brain being involved in Alzheimer's disease includes abnormalities in red blood cells (RBCs), lymphocytes, polymorphonuclear leukocytes, platelets, and fibroblasts. These cells have been investigated for a number of different reasons (e.g., RBCs because they have virtues as model membranes and their low-affinity choline transport mechanism resembles that of cholinergic nerve terminals), but primarily because they can be obtained from living individuals in a relatively nonstressful way.

The findings of nonneural cell abnormalities fit well within the postulate of genetic factors in the etiology of Alzheimer's disease. Since DNA is present, at some time, in all cells of the body, the possibility that the abnormal gene(s) may be expressed in cells other than brain cells may account for the abnormal findings in a variety of tissues.

Third Prediction

The specific vulnerabilities—whether inherited or acquired—*will remain hidden until exposed by appropriate stressors.* For example, an individual may be endowed with fewer then the normal complement of a certain type of nerve cell (i.e., cholinergic or adrenergic, producing somatostatin or corticotropin releasing factor), but the abnormality will not appear until the supply of these nerve cells is further reduced by disease, trauma, toxins, or age-associated losses—or until circumstances demand more than the usual level of activity from such cells. That is the threshold phenomenon described by Sir Martin Roth many years ago (Roth et al., 1967).

Fourth Prediction

The specific individual vulnerabilities will lead to identification of specific means of intervention and prevention. For example, an impairment in acetylcholine metabolism leading to the inadequate levels of acetylcholine that have been implicated in the memory loss so characteristic of Alzheimer's disease suggests several treatment approaches. Dietary supplements (e.g., lecithin) can be bought in health-food stores, but unfortunately, their composition varies widely. Even with the purified lecithin compound (i.e., known phosphatidylcholine content), the results have so far not been promising (Bartus et al., 1982). Nonetheless, nutritional factors may be critical in the etiology and pathogenesis of Alzheimer's disease (Wurtman, 1985a). Another approach attempts to slow the breakdown of acetylcholine so that there will be more acetylcholine available and its level will decrease more slowly. Physostigmine has been used for this purpose (Mohs et al., 1985) since it inhibits the enzyme acetylcholinesterase, which breaks down acetylcholine.

Tetrahydroaminoacridine (tacrin or THA) is the latest and purportedly most potent entry into the field (Summers et al., 1981, 1986); the reported results await replication, and a clinical trial is currently in the planning phase. Other approaches include brain transplants of cholinergic cells, as pioneered in animals by Cotman and associates (Geddes et al., 1985)—perhaps not much more heroic than the infusion pump for the delivery of bethanechol directly into the brain ventricles, which is currently in vogue (Harbaugh et al., 1984), or adrenergic supplements as pioneered in rhesus monkeys (Arnsten & Goldman-Rakic, 1985).

Areas of brain deficits may be identified with sophisticated imaging technologies that will be the successors to positron emission tomography (PET) scanning (Phelps & Mazziotta, 1985; Holman et al., 1985). Different treatments will be effective for different individuals, depending upon the particular deficit(s) characteristic for each. Some defects may require genetic engineering; some (e.g., immune disorders) may respond to treatment with interleukin-2 (Thoman, 1985); others to treatment with estrogens (H. J. Weinreb, Rockefeller University, personal communication, 1986); and still others may require careful fine-tuning of neurotransmitter balances. I will let your imagination conjure up the rest.

THE FUTURE HOLDS PROMISE

Do these predictions sound too simplistic? They probably are. But they have served their purpose if they lead us to fruitful research. After all, we learn from our errors far more often than we learn from our successes. Karl Lashley, for example, one of our most famous neuroscientists, spent many a year in futile attempts to localize brain sites corresponding to behavior. Finally, he concluded that the only reasonable interpretation of his experimental results was: there is no such thing as learning. Since he knew better than to accept that conclusion, he formulated the law of mass action, which reigned for decades—until a new generation with much more sophisticated technology has now embarked on another search for the engram! Lashley's example can be matched in every field of science—over and over again.

Let me cite just one more illustration—for which I am indebted to Isaac Asimov and my airline magazine, our jet-age source of scientific information. Christopher Columbus tried in vain to convince the Portuguese that instead of sailing to India by going east around Africa, a voyage of some 10,000 miles, he could get there by sailing west some 3,000 miles. The Portuguese geographers refused to accept his calculations; their own showed it to be the longer, not the shorter route. Had Columbus not been wrong, had he known that in truth 12,000 westward miles separated him from Asia, he would not have made the trip. And where would we be today?

Enough speculation about the past. To turn again to the future, I am optimistic that before this millenium comes to a close, we will have found treatments effective for Alzheimer's disease—treatments to cure and treatments to prevent the disease. Let us hope that my optimism is well-founded. By the year 2000 we expect over 17 million Americans in the age group 75 years and older. At current rates, that would mean 3.5 million victims of Alzheimer's disease, not a situation to which I want to look forward. Instead, I would like to see our centenarians of the twenty-first century be as alert as one of the survivors from our twin study, who wrote us the following letter in her own nontremulous handwriting four months before her 100th birthday.

"I am interested in the Cosmos which is shown on TV by Carl Sagan. I find so many new inventions which are not fully distributed which I will have to study, also will destroy the World. Happy to hear from you. Sincerely."

Grant support from: NIMH Research Grant MH36205 and the Veterans Administration. The opinions expressed herein are those of the author and not necessarily those of the Veterans Administration.

Epilogue

Robert N. Butler

What, after all, is Alzheimer's disease? Is it a disease, or, as I believe, a group of diseases? Is it neurologic? Is it psychiatric? It is a disease we cannot actually diagnose and cannot cure. We know very little about it, although we now talk a great deal about it. We can only study it with great difficulty. We cannot precisely identify it or measure its severity, and we have no available animal models. Because we have no established measures, its epidemiology is poorly understood.

To the degree to which the disease is the result of neuronal damage, we cannot at this stage do anything about it. To the degree to which it manifests itself in behavioral, psychiatric symptoms, we can intervene.

We know so little of this disease, yet it is, as Lewis Thomas has said, "the disease of the century" (Thomas, 1981). Especially for the growing number of people over 85, the risk of developing Alzheimer's disease is great—a chance of approximately 20%. Research data suggest that in some families (proportion unknown) this disease may be caused by an autosomal dominant gene with late-life penetrance. Thus the increasing average life expectancy will lead to increasing prevalence in the future. By the time the baby-boomers reach "golden pond" in their eighties, circa 2020, there may be 4 million people with Alzheimer's disease, and 4 million people (many with Alzheimer's disease) will reside in nursing homes (there is a large overlap between these two populations).

Unfortunately for those afflicted, Alzheimer's disease is considered incurable and, therefore, untreatable. This results in an attitude of therapeutic nihilism on the part of many professionals. Coupled with prejudice against the aged and scarce resources, this nihilism leads to warehousing of "senile" patients, as the disease progresses, and the manifestations of dementia make the patient both unattractive and disturbing to us all. Yet Alzheimer's disease *is* treatable.

Despite the need to establish Alzheimer's disease as a major social and medical priority, and the strong efforts of many to do so, funding for research, training, treatment, and education remains grossly inadequate. FY 1986 federal money allotted for research was $61 million. This hardly constitutes a true national priority. By contrast, the National Cancer Institute receives well over $1 billion per year of well-deserved funding. Cancer is the third most prevalent disease in the United States, while Alzheimer's disease is number four. Obviously, something is out of balance.

One might, however, question why money should be provided for a disease, no matter how serious and widespread, if there is little hope for discovering a cure. But there is hope. The neurosciences are flourishing. Some 50 of the probable 200 neurotransmitters are now known. It seems now that Alzheimer's disease is a multineurotransmitter deficiency rather than a single deficiency. But even a complex model of multiple deficiencies is not enough. Research is needed that will consider the possibility that these phenomena, though significant, may nonetheless be epiphenomena that cover up other underlying chemical abnormalities.

New technologies and instrumentation are now available to aid us in clinical research. In addition to computerized axial tomography, there is position emission tomography (PET) and magnetic resonance imaging. We have already gained knowledge about metabolism in Alzheimer's disease from PET scanning. Moreover, the new biology illustrated by recombinant DNA (gene splicing) makes possible work at the molecular level that may lead to the unraveling of central nervous system dysfunctions that underlie Alzheimer's disease.

Furthermore, there are other suggestive findings regarding Alzheimer's disease that may prove valuable to our understanding of the disease. For example, in the terrible plague AIDS, dementia also occurs. Research into Alzheimer's-related dementia may uncover a link with the AIDS retrovirus. Head trauma, also, may have a relationship to the development of Alzheimer's disease in late life, and this lead must be pursued.

Other avenues of research are also under exploration. Amyloid (resembling starch), an interesting abnormal chemical (most probably a glycoprotein), is found in the core of the neuritic plaque. Believed to contain antigen–antibody complexes, it requires major study, since this suggests the possibility of an infectious basis for Alzheimer's disease.

But what is to be done until our government makes Alzheimer's research a true priority? What is to be done until there are research breakthroughs that make cure a possibility? The answer is that while waiting we must treat, and we must treat actively. Alzheimer's disease primary pathology, brain damage—which causes disorientation, confusion, memory loss, and intellectual dysfunction—is not currently reversible, but its clinical manifestations can be temporarily improved through reorientation exercises. Secondary symptoms (excess disabilities of Alzheimer's disease such as depression, malnutrition, insomnia, and incontinence) are, indeed, treatable and manageable. Since the central nervous system affects all aspects of psychological and social adjustment, treatment of secondary symptoms will alleviate considerable suffering. Patients who may not be able to remember when to eat or when to take medications need careful supervision and nursing care. Appropriate stimuli in the environment can help maintain the patient's functioning and prevent the irritability and anxiety that ensue when patients are confronted with challenges they cannot meet. Judicious use of medication can reduce depression, anxiety, and hostility. Counseling of patients and their families should include guidance about legal, financial, and safety matters as well as emotional issues. Geriatric counseling may be helpful. Support groups and information from the national Alzheimer's Disease and Related Disorders Association can also be extremely beneficial to Alzheimer families. Most important, treatment should be focused on maintaining the dignity and respect of the patient by maximizing the privacy, freedom, and identity of the Alzheimer sufferer. For the goals of quality treatment to be met, society will have to alter the financial policies that inflict great punishment on Alzheimer victims and their families.

The capacity of VA facilities to provide adequate care for eligible Alzheimer victims must be enhanced. Medicare must be restructured to provide for elderly patients who require long-term, multifaceted care rather than brief periods of assistance for acute illness. The great critical need in health services is increasingly in long-term care, both institutional and noninstitutional. Access and quality vie constantly with cost. When costs are reduced, so, usually, are access or quality or both.

Yet the restructuring of Medicare might be possible with relatively little increase in cost (other than that required by the increasing number of older persons) through rationalizing the system, using paraprofessionals, and introducing prevention, rehabilitation, and long-term care.

To address the health needs of the surging population of elderly, and hence of Alzheimer patients, we must speak, finally, of ethical and cultural values. Unless we can counter the growing materialism of our culture and the increasing commercialization of the health care system, the likelihood is that many, particularly the poor, and most especially older women, will be left out in the cold.

What does the future hold? Basic research holds the greatest hope for cost containment and even cure. According to Lewis Thomas, we cannot predict the course of scientific discovery, even when it is adequately funded (Thomas, 1985). But we can predict that without governmental support for basic research, Alzheimer's disease will remain the great, and expensive, scourge of old age, tainting with fear our view of growing old.

Appendices

Appendix 1
Mini-Mental
State Examination

This scale must be administered by a trained professional. It cannot be used to make a diagnosis, but is useful for following patient changes over time. Variations in scores occur as a result of many factors (e.g., fatigue, coexistent illness, medications). Therefore, a single score cannot be clinically definitive. Since scores are most appropriately used for research purposes, the scoring criteria are not included here.

I. Orientation (Maximum score 10)
Ask "What is today's date?" Then ask specifically for parts omitted: e.g., "Can you also tell me what season it is?"

Date (e.g., January 21)	1 __
Year	2 __
Month	3 __
Day (e.g., Monday) ..	4 __
Season	5 __

Ask
"Can you tell me the name of this hospital?"
"What floor are we on?"
"What town (or city) are we in?"
"What county are we in?"
"What state are we in?"

Hospital	6 __
Floor	7 __
Town/City	8 __
County	9 __
State	10 __

II. Registration (Maximum score 3)
Ask the subject if you may test his/her memory. Then say "ball," "flag," "tree" clearly and slowly, about one second for each. After you have said all 3 words, ask subject to repeat them. This first repetition determines the score (0–3), but keep saying them (up to 6 trials) until the subject can repeat all 3 words. If (s)he does not eventually learn all three, recall cannot be meaningfully tested

"ball"	11 __
"flag"	12 __
"tree"	13 __

Record number of trials: __

III. Attention and calculation (Maximum score 5)
Ask the subject to begin at 100 and count backward by 7. Stop after 5 subtractions

"93"	14 __
"86"	15 __

(continued)

(93, 86, 79, 72, 65). Score one point for each correct number

"79" .... 16 —
"72" .... 17 —
"65" .... 18 —
OR

If the subject cannot or will not perform this task, ask him/her to spell the word "world" backwards (D, L, R, O, W). The score is one point for each correctly placed letter, e.g., DLROW = 5, DLORW = 3. Record how the subject spelled "world" backwards:

Number of correctly-placed letters .... 19 —

D L R O W

IV. Recall (Maximum score 3)
Ask the subject to recall the three words you previously asked him/her to remember (learned in Registration)

"ball" .... 20 —
"flag" .... 21 —
"tree" .... 22 —

V. Language (Maximum score 9)
Naming: Show the subject a wrist watch and ask "What is this?" Repeat for pencil. Score one point for each item named correctly

Watch .... 23 —
Pencil .... 24 —

Repetition: Ask the subject to repeat, "No ifs, ands, or buts." Score one point for correct repetition

Repetition .... 25 —

3-Stage Command: Give the subject a piece of blank paper and say, "Take the paper in your right hand, fold it in half and put in on the floor." Score one point for each action performed correctly

Takes in right hand . 26 —
Folds in half .... 27 —
Puts on floor .... 28 —

Reading: On a blank piece of paper, print the sentence "Close your eyes" in letters large enough for the subject to see clearly. Ask subject to read it and do what it says. Score correct only if (s)he actually closes his/her eyes

Closes eyes .... 29 —

Writing: Give the subject a blank piece of paper and ask him/her to write a sentence. It is to be written spontaneously. It must contain a subject and verb and make sense. Correct grammar and punctuation are not necessary

Writes sentence .... 30 —

(*continued*)

Copying: On a clean piece of paper
draw intersecting pentagons, each side
about 1 inch, and ask subject to copy it
exactly as it is. All 10 angles must be
present and two must intersect to score
1 point. Tremor and rotation are   Draws pentagons ...... 31 __
ignored E.g.,

Score: Add number of correct responses. In
       section III include items 14–18 or item 19,
       not both. (Maximum total score 30)

                                                            Total score ____

Rate subject's level of consciousness:
_____ (a) coma, (b) stupor, (c) drowsy, (d) alert

Source: Reprinted with permission from *J. Psychiatr. Res.* 12(3):189, M.F. Folstein, S. E.
Folstein, and P. R. McHugh, "'Mini-Mental State': A Practical Method for Grading the
Cognitive State of Patients for the Clinician." Copyright 1975, Pergamon Press, Ltd.

Appendix 2
Clinical Dementia
Rating (CDR) Scale

This scale must be administered by a trained professional. It cannot be used to make a diagnosis, but is useful for following patient changes over time. Variations in scores occur as a result of many factors (e.g., fatigue, coexistent illness, medications). Therefore, a single score cannot be clinically definitive. Since scores are most appropriately used for research purposes, the scoring criteria are not included here.

Impairment:	None	Questionable	Mild	Moderate	Severe
MEMORY	No memory loss or slight inconstant forgetfulness	Consistent slight forgetfulness; partial recollection of events; "benign" forgetfulness	Moderate memory loss; more marked for recent events; defect interferes with everyday activities	Severe memory loss; only highly learned material retained; new material rapidly lost	Severe memory loss; only fragments remain
ORIENTA-TION	Fully oriented	Fully oriented except for slight difficulty with time relationships	Moderate difficulty with time relationships; oriented for place at examination; may have geographic disorientation elsewhere	Severe difficulty with time relationships; usually disoriented in time, often to place	Oriented to person only

JUDGMENT + PROBLEM SOLVING	Solves everyday problems well; judgment good in relation to past performance	Slight impairment in solving problems, similarities, differences	Moderate difficulty in handling problems, similarities, differences; social judgment usually maintained	Severely impaired in handling problems, similarities, differences; social judgment usually impaired	Unable to make judgments or solve problems
COMMUNITY AFFAIRS	Independent function at usual level in job, shopping, business and financial affairs, volunteer and social groups	Slight impairment in these activities	Unable to function independently at these activities though may still be engaged in some; appears normal to casual inspection	No pretense of independent function outside home. Appears well enough to be taken to functions outside a family home	No pretense of independent function outside home. Appears too ill to be taken to functions outside a family home
HOME + HOBBIES	Life at home, hobbies, intellectual interests well maintained	Life at home, hobbies, intellectual interests slightly impaired	Mild but definite impairment of function at home; more difficult chores abandoned; more complicated hobbies and interests abandoned	Only simple chores preserved; very restricted interests, poorly sustained	No significant function in home
PERSONAL CARE	Fully capable of self-care		Needs prompting	Requires assistance in dressing, hygiene, keeping of personal effects	Requires much help with personal care; frequent incontinence

Score only as decline from previous usual level due to cognitive loss, not impairment due to other factors.

Source: From Mild Senile dementia of the Alzheimer type: Diagnostic criteria and natural history by L. Berg, 1988. In TS Elizan (Ed.), Alzheimer's and Parkinson's Diseases and The Aging Brain, *Mt. Sinai J Med*, 55, p. 87. Copyright 1988. Reprinted by permission.

Appendix 3
Index of Independence
in Activities of
Daily Living

This scale must be administered by a trained professional. It cannot be used to make a diagnosis, but is useful for following patient changes over time. Variations in scores occur as a result of many factors (e.g., fatigue, coexistent illness, medications). Therefore, a single score cannot be clinically definitive. Since scores are most appropriately used for research purposes, the scoring criteria are not included here.

The Index of Independence in Activities of Daily Living is based on an evaluation of the functional independence or dependence of patients in bathing, dressing, going to the toilet, transferring, continence, and feeding. Specific definitions of functional independence and dependence appear below the index.

A   Independent in feeding, continence, transferring, going to toilet, dressing, and bathing.

B   Independent in all but one of these functions.

C   Independent in all but bathing and one additional function.

D   Independent in all but bathing, dressing, and one additional function.

E   Independent in all but bathing, dressing, going to toilet, and one additional function.

F   Independent in all but bathing, dressing, going to toilet, transferring, and one additional function.

G   Dependent in all six functions.

Other   Dependent in at least two functions, but not classifiable as C, D, E, or F.

Independence means without supervision, direction, or active personal assistance, except as specifically noted below. This is based on actual status and not on ability. A patient who refuses to perform a function is considered as not performing the function, even though he is deemed able.

Bathing (Sponge, shower, or tub)
Independent: assistance only in bathing a single part (as back or disabled extremity) or bathes self completely
Dependent: assistance in bathing more

Transfer
Independent: moves in and out of bed independently and moves in and out of chair independently (may or may not be using mechanical supports)

(*continued*)

than one part of body; assistance in getting in or out of tub or does not bathe self

Dependent: assistance in moving in or out of bed and/or chair; does not perform one or more transfers

Dressing
Independent: gets clothes from closets and drawers; puts on clothes, outer garments, braces; manages fasteners; act of tying shoes is excluded
Dependent: does not dress self or remains partly undressed

Continence
Independent: urination and defecation entirely self-controlled
Dependent: partial or total incontinence in urination or defecation; partial or total control by enemas, catheters, or regulated use of urinals and/or bedpans

Going to toilet
Independent: gets to toilet; gets on and off toilet; arranges clothes, cleans organs of excretion; (may manage own bedpan used at night only and may or may not be using mechanical supports)
Dependent: uses bedpan or commode or receives assistance in getting to and using toilet

Feeding
Independent: gets food from plate or its equivalent into mouth; (precutting of meat and preparation of food, as buttering bread, are excluded from evaluation).
Dependent: assistance in act of feeding (see above); does not eat at all or parenteral feeding.

EVALUATION FORM

Name _____ Date of Evaluation _____

For each area of functioning listed below, check description that applies. (The word *assistance* means supervision, direction, or personal assistance.)

Bathing—either sponge bath, tub bath, or shower

☐ Receives no assistance (gets in and out of tub by self if tub is usual means of bathing)

☐ Receives assistance in bathing only one part of body (such as back or a leg)

☐ Receives assistance in bathing more than one part of body (or not bathed)

Dressing—gets clothes from closets and drawers—including underclothes, outer garments, and using fasteners (including braces, if worn)

☐ Gets clothes and gets completely dressed without assistance

☐ Gets clothes and gets dressed without assistance except for assistance in tying shoes

☐ Receives assistance in getting clothes or in getting dressed, or stays partly or completely undressed

(*continued*)

Toileting—going to the "toilet room" for bowel and urine elimination; cleaning self after elimination and arranging clothes

☐	☐	☐
Goes to "toilet room," cleans self, and arranges clothes without assistance (may use object for support such as cane, walker, or wheelchair and may manage night bedpan or commode, emptying same in morning)	Receives assistance in going to "toilet room" or in cleansing self or in arranging clothes after elimination or in use of night bedpan or commode	Doesn't go to room termed "toilet" for the elimination process

Transfer—

☐	☐	☐
Moves in and out of bed as well as in and out of chair without assistance (may be using object for support such as cane or walker)	Moves in or out of bed or chair with assistance	Doesn't get out of bed

Continence—

☐	☐	☐
Controls urination and bowel movement completely by self	Has occasional "accidents"	Supervision helps keep urine or bowel control; catheter is used or is incontinent

Feeding—

☐	☐	☐
Feeds self without assistance	Feeds self except for getting assistance in cutting meat or buttering bread	Receives assistance in feeding or is fed partly or completely by using tubes or intravenous fluids

Source: S. Katz, T.D. Downs, H.R. Cash, and R.C. Grotz, 1970. Reprinted by permission of *The Gerontologist,* Vol. 10, No.1, Spring 1970.

Appendix 4
Physical Self-Maintenance Scale

This scale must be administered by a trained professional. It cannot be used to make a diagnosis, but is useful for following patient changes over time. Variations in scores occur as a result of many factors (e.g., fatigue, coexistent illness, medications). Therefore, a single score cannot be clinically definitive. Since scores are most appropriately used for research purposes, the scoring criteria are not included here.

Circle one statement in each category A–F that applies to subject.

Scoring: Score 1 for first statement in each category, 0 for all other statements. Score 9 for missing data.

A. Toilet
   1. Cares for self at toilet completely, no incontinence
   2. Needs to be reminded or needs help in cleaning self, or has rare (weekly at most) accidents
   3. Soiling or wetting while asleep more than once a week
   4. Soiling or wetting while awake more than once a week
   5. No control of bowels or bladder

Score _____

B. Feeding
   1. Eats without assistance
   2. Eats with minor assistance at meal times and/or with special preparation of food, or help in cleaning up after meals
   3. Feeds self with moderate assistance and is untidy
   4. Requires extensive assistance for all meals
   5. Does not feed self at all and resists efforts of others to feed him/her

Score _____

(continued)

C. Dressing
    1. Dresses, undresses, and selects clothes from own wardrobe
    2. Dresses and undresses self with minor assistance
    3. Needs moderate assistance in dressing or selection of clothes
    4. Needs major assistance in dressing but cooperates with efforts of others to help
    5. Completely unable to dress self and resists efforts of others to help

Score _____

D. Grooming (neatness, hair, nails, hands, face, clothing)
    1. Always neatly dressed, well groomed, without assistance
    2. Grooms self adequately with occasional minor assistance, e.g., shaving
    3. Needs moderate and regular assistance or supervision in grooming
    4. Needs total grooming care, but can remain well groomed after help from others
    5. Actively negates all efforts of others to maintain grooming

Score _____

E. Physical Ambulation
    1. Goes about grounds or city
    2. Ambulates within residence or about one block distant
    3. Ambulates with assistance of (check one):
        a. another person
        b. railing
        c. cane
        d. walker
        e. wheelchair
    4. Sits unsupported in chair or wheelchair but cannot propel self without help
    5. Bedridden more than half the time

Score _____

F. Bathing
    1. Bathes self (tub, shower, sponge bath) without help
    2. Bathes self with help in getting in and out of tub
    3. Washes face and hands only, but cannot bathe rest of body
    4. Does not wash self but is cooperative with those who bathe him/her

5. Does not try to wash self and resists efforts to keep
   him/her clean

Score _____

Total Score _____
(0–6)

Source: M.P. Lawton and E.M. Brody, 1969. Reprinted by permission of the *The Geronto-logist*, Vol. 9, No. 3, Autumn 1969.

Appendix 5
Instrumental Activities of Daily Living Scale

This scale must be administered by a trained professional. It cannot be used to make a diagnosis, but is useful for following patient changes over time. Variations in scores occur as a result of many factors (e.g., fatigue, coexistent illness, medications). Therefore, a single score cannot be clinically definitive. Since scores are most appropriately used for research purposes, the scoring criteria are not included here.

Scoring: Score each statement as indicated in parentheses. Score 9 for missing data.

Circle one statement in each category A–H that applies to subject.

A. Ability to use telephone
   1. Operates telephone on own initiative—looks up and dials numbers, etc.   (1)
   2. Dials a few well-known numbers   (1)
   3. Answers telephone, but does not dial   (1)
   4. Does not use telephone at all   (0)

Score_____

B. Shopping
   1. Takes care of all shopping needs independently   (1)
   2. Shops independently for small purchases   (0)
   3. Needs to be accompanied on any shopping trip   (0)
   4. Completely unable to shop   (0)

Score_____

C. Food preparation
   1. Plans, prepares, and serves adequate meals independently   (1)
   2. Prepares adequate meals if supplied with ingredients   (0)
   3. Heats and serves prepared meals, or prepares meals but does not maintain adequate diet   (0)
   4. Needs to have meals prepared and served   (0)

Score_____

(continued)

D. Housekeeping
   1. Maintains house alone or with occasional assistance (e.g., "heavy-work-domestic help")   (1)
   2. Performs light daily tasks such as dishwashing, bedmaking   (1)
   3. Performs light daily tasks but cannot maintain acceptable levels of cleanliness   (1)
   4. Needs help with all home-maintenance tasks   (1)
   5. Does not participate in any housekeeping tasks   (0)

   Score＿＿＿＿＿

E. Laundry
   1. Does personal laundry completely   (1)
   2. Launders small items—rinses socks, stockings, etc.   (1)
   3. All laundry must be done by others   (0)

   Score ＿＿＿＿＿

F. Mode of transportation
   1. Travels independently on public transportation or drives own car   (1)
   2. Arranges own travel via taxi, but does not otherwise use public transportation   (1)
   3. Travels on public transportation when assisted or accompanied by another   (1)
   4. Travel limited to taxi or automobile with assistance of another   (0)
   5. Does not travel at all   (0)

   Score＿＿＿＿＿

G. Responsibility for own medications
   1. Is responsible for taking medication in correct dosages at correct time   (1)
   2. Takes responsibility if medication is prepared in advance in separate dosages   (0)
   3. Is not capable of dispensing own medication   (0)

   Score＿＿＿＿＿

H. Ability to handle finances
   1. Manages financial matters independently (budgets, writes checks, pays rent, bills, goes to bank)   (1)
   2. Manages day-to-day purchases but needs help with banking, major purchases, etc.   (1)
   3. Incapable of handling money   (0)

   Score ＿＿＿＿＿
   Total Score ＿＿＿＿＿

Source: M. P. Lawton and E. M. Brody, 1969. Reprinted by permission of *The Gerontologist,* Vol. 9, No. 3, Autumn 1969.

Appendix 6
Geriatric Depression
Scale (Short Form)

This scale is usually self administered. However, a clinician may need to help some patients, especially those who are cognitively impaired. Sometimes patients fail to notice that some questions are worded positively and others negatively. This scale cannot be used to make a diagnosis, but is useful for following patient changes over time. Variations in scores occur as a result of many factors (e.g., fatigue, coexistent illness, medications). Therefore, a single score cannot be clinically definitive. Since scores are most appropriately used for research purposes, the scoring criteria are not included here.

Choose the best answer for how you felt over the past week

1.	Are you basically satisfied with your life?	yes / no
2.	Have you dropped many of your activities and interests?	yes / no
3.	Do you feel that your life is empty?	yes / no
4.	Do you often get bored?	yes / no
5.	Are you in good spirits most of the time?	yes / no
6.	Are you afraid that something bad is going to happen to you?	yes / no
7.	Do you feel happy most of the time?	yes / no
8.	Do you often feel helpless?	yes / no
9.	Do you prefer to stay at home, rather than going out and doing new things?	yes / no
10.	Do you feel you have more problems with memory than most?	yes / no
11.	Do you think it is wonderful to be alive now?	yes / no
12.	Do you feel pretty worthless the way you are now?	yes / no
13.	Do you feel full of energy?	yes / no
14.	Do you feel that your situation is hopeless?	yes / no
15.	Do you think that most people are better off than you are?	yes / no

The following "no" answers count one point (1, 5, 7, 11, and 13);
The remaining yes answers count 1 point.
Scores > 5 indicate probable depression.

Source: From "Geriatric Depression Scale (GDS) Recent Evidence and Development of a shorter version" by J.L. Sheikh and J.A. Yesavage, 1986, *Clinical Gerontologist*, 5, p. 165. Copyright 1986 by Haworth Press, Inc., 12 West 32nd St., New York, NY 10001. Adapted by permission.

Appendix 7
Hamilton Psychiatric Rating Scale for Depression

This scale must be administered by a trained professional. It cannot be used to make a diagnosis, but is useful for following patient changes over time. Variations in scores occur as a result of many factors (e.g., fatigue, coexistent illness, medications). Therefore, a single score cannot be clinically definitive. Since scores are most appropriately used for research purposes, the scoring criteria are not included here.

1. Depressed mood (Sadness, hopeless, helpless, worthless)	0	Absent
	1	These feeling states indicated only on questioning
	2	These feeling states spontaneously reported verbally
	3	Communicates feeling states nonverbally—i.e., through facial expression, posture, voice, and tendency to weep
	4	Patient reports *virtually only* these feeling states in his spontaneous verbal and nonverbal communication
2. Feelings of guilt	0	Absent
	1	Self-reproach, feels he has let people down
	2	Ideas of guilt or rumination over past errors or sinful deeds
	3	Present illness is a punishment; delusions of guilt
	4	Hears accusatory or denunciatory voices and/or experiences threatening visual hallucinations
3. Suicide	0	Absent
	1	Feels life is not worth living
	2	Wishes he were dead or any thoughts of possible death to self
	3	Suicide ideas or gesture
	4	Attempts at suicide (any serious attempt rates 4)
4. Insomnia—early	0	No difficulty falling asleep
	1	Complaints of occasional difficulty falling asleep—i.e., more than one-half hour
	2	Complaints of nightly difficulty falling asleep

(continued)

5. Insomnia— middle	0	No difficulty
	1	Patient complains of being restless and disturbed during the night
	2	Waking during the night—any getting out of bed rates 2 (except for purposes of voiding)

6. Insomnia—late	0	No difficulty
	1	Waking in early hours of the morning but goes back to sleep
	2	Unable to fall asleep again if gets out of bed

7. Work and activities	0	No difficulty
	1	Thoughts and feelings of incapacity, fatigue, or weakness related to activities, work, or hobbies
	2	Loss of interest in activity, hobbies, or work— either directly reported by patient, or indirect in listlessness, indecision, and vacillation (feels he has to push self to work or join activities)
	3	Decrease in actual time spent in activities or decrease in productivity; in hospital, rate 3 if patient does not spend at least three hours a day in activities (hospital job or hobbies) exclusive of ward chores
	4	Stopped working because of present illness; in hospital, rate 4 if patient engages in no activities except ward chores, or if patient fails to perform ward chores unassisted

8. Retardation (Slowness of thought and speech; impaired ability to concentrate; decreased motor activity)	0	Normal speech and thought
	1	Slight retardation at interview
	2	Obvious retardation at interview
	3	Interview difficult
	4	Complete stupor

9. Agitation	0	None
	1	Fidgetiness
	2	"Playing with" hands, hair, etc.
	3	Moving about, can't sit still
	4	Hand-wringing, nail-biting, hair-pulling, biting of lips

10. Anxiety— psychic	0	No difficulty
	1	Subjective tension and irritability
	2	Worrying about minor matters
	3	Apprehensive attitude apparent in face or speech
	4	Fears expressed without questioning

(*continued*)

11. Anxiety—
    somatic

0	Absent	Physiological concomitants of anxiety, such as:
1	Mild	Gastrointestinal—dry mouth, wind,
2	Moderate	indigestion, diarrhea, cramps, belching
3	Severe	Cardiovascular—palpitations, headaches
4	Incapacitating	Respiratory—hyperventilation, sighing
		Urinary frequency
		Sweating

12. Somatic symp-
    toms—
    gastrointestinal

0 None
1 Loss of appetite but eating without staff encouragement; heavy feelings in abdomen
2 Difficulty eating without staff urging; requests or requires laxatives or medication for bowels or medication for GI symptoms.

13. Somatic symp-
    toms—general

0 None
1 Heaviness in limbs, back, or head; backaches, headache, muscle aches; loss of energy and fatigability
2 Any clear-cut symptom rates 2

14. Genital symp-
    toms

0	Absent	Symptoms such as:	Loss of libido
1	Mild		Menstrual dis-
2	Severe		turbances

15. Hypochondriasis

0 Not present
1 Self-absorption (bodily)
2 Preoccupation with health
3 Frequent complaints, requests for help, etc.
4 Hypochondriacal delusions

16. Loss of weight

Rating by history:
0 No weight loss
1 Probable weight loss associated with present illness
2 Definite (according to patient) weight loss
3 Not assessed

17. Insight

0 Acknowledges being depressed and ill
1 Acknowledges illness but attributes cause to bad food, climate, overwork, virus, need for rest, etc.
2 Denies being ill at all

(*continued*)

18. Diurnal varia-   Note whether symptoms are worse in the morning or
    tion   evening. If *no* diurnal variation, mark "no variation"
                         0   No variation
                         1   Worse in morning
                               —Severity of the variation: 0 = None
                               1 = Mild   2 = Severe
                         2   Worse in evening

19. Depersonaliza-   0   Absent
    tion and de-   1   Mild   Such as: Feelings of unreality
    realization   Nihilistic ideas
                         2   Moderate
                         3   Severe
                         4   Incapacitating

20. Paranoid symp-   0   None
    toms   1   Suspicious
                         2   Ideas of reference
                         3   Delusions of reference and persecution

21. Obsessional and   0   Absent
    compulsive   1   Mild
    symptoms   2   Severe

Source: From "A Rating Scale for Depression" by M. Hamilton, 1960, *Journal of Neurology, Neurosurgery and Psychiatry,* 23, p. 56. Copyright 1960 by British Medical Journal. Reprinted by permission.

Appendix 8
Zung Self-Rating Depression Scale

This scale is usually self administered. However, a clinician may need to help some patients, especially those who are cognitively impaired. Sometimes patients fail to notice that some questions are worded positively and others negatively. This scale cannot be used to make a diagnosis, but is useful for following patient changes over time. Variations in scores occur as a result of many factors (e.g., fatigue, coexistent illness, medications). Therefore, a single score cannot be clinically definitive. Since scores are most appropriately used for research purposes, the scoring criteria are not included here.

Please circle the X under the appropriate column:	None or a little of the time	Some of the time	Good part of the time	Most or all of the time
1. I feel down-hearted, blue, and sad.	X	X	X	X
2. Morning is when I feel the best.	X	X	X	X
3. I have crying spells or feel like it.	X	X	X	X
4. I have trouble sleeping through the night.	X	X	X	X
5. I eat as much as I used to.	X	X	X	X
6. I enjoy looking at, talking to, and being with attractive women/men.	X	X	X	X
7. I notice that I am losing weight.	X	X	X	X
8. I have trouble with constipation.	X	X	X	X
9. My heart beats faster than usual.	X	X	X	X
10. I get tired for no reason.	X	X	X	X
11. My mind is as clear as it used to be.	X	X	X	X
12. I find it easy to do the things I used to.	X	X	X	X
13. I am restless and can't keep still.	X	X	X	X
14. I feel hopeful about the future.	X	X	X	X
15. I am more irritable than usual.	X	X	X	X
16. I find it easy to make decisions.	X	X	X	X
17. I feel that I am useful and needed.	X	X	X	X
18. My life is pretty full.	X	X	X	X
19. I feel that others would be better off if I were dead.	X	X	X	X
20. I still enjoy the things I used to do.	X	X	X	X

Source: From "A Self-Rating Depression Scale" by W. Zung, 1965, *Archives of General Psychiatry*, 12, p. 63. Copyright 1965 by American Medical Association. Reprinted by permission.

References

Abse DW, Dahlstrom WG. The value of chemotherapy in senile mental disturbance. Controlled comparison of chlorpromazine, reserpine-pipradol, and opium. *JAMA* 1960; 174:2036–2042.

Albert MS, Moss M. The assessment of memory disorders in patients with Alzheimer disease. In LR Squire, N Butters (eds.), *Neuropsychology of Memory*. New York: Guilford Press, 1984, pp. 236–246.

Alexopoulos GS, Lieberman KW, Young RC. Platelet MAO activity in primary degenerative dementia. *Am J Psychiatry* 1984; 141(1):97–99.

Allan C, Brotman H. *Chartbook on Aging in America*. (Compiled for the 1981 White House Conference on Aging.) Washington, DC: U.S. Government Printing Office, 1981.

Alzheimer A. Uber eine eigenartige Erkrankung der Hirnrinde. *Allgemeine Zeitschrift fur Psychiatrie und Psychische Medizin* 1907; 64:146–148.

Amaducci LA, Fratiglioni L, Rocca WA, Fieschi C, Livrea P, Pedone D, Bracco L, Lippi A, Gandolfo C, Bino G, Prencipe M, Bonatti ML, Girotti F, Carella F, Tavolato B, Ferla S, Lenzi GL, Carolei A, Gambi A, Grigoletto F, Schoenberg BS. Risk factors for clinically diagnosed Alzheimer's disease: A case-control study of an Italian population. *Neurology* 1986; 36(7):922–931.

The American Dietetic Association. *Handbook of Clinical Dietetics*. New Haven: Yale University Press, 1981, pp. 17–21.

American Drug Index, 31st Edition. Philadelphia: J.B. Lippincott, 1987.

American Hospital Farmulary Service. *Drug Information 1987*. Bethesda, MD: American Society of Hospital Pharmacists, 1987.

American Medical Association, Council on Scientific Affairs. Dementia. *JAMA* 1986; 256(16):2234–2238.

American Psychiatric Association, Task Force on Nomenclature and Statistics. *Diagnostic and Statistical Manual of Mental Disorders, Third Edition, Revised* (DSM-III-R). Washington, DC: American Psychiatric Association, 1987.

Anderson GF. National medical care spending. *Health Aff* 1985; 4(3):100–107.

Andia-Waltenbaugh AM, Puck TT. Alzheimer's disease: Further evidence of a microtubular defect [abstract]. *J Cell Biol* 1977; 75(2, Part 2):279a.

Anthony JC, LeResche L, Niaz U, von Korff MR, Folstein MF. Limits of the 'Mini-Mental State' as a screening test for dementia and delirium among hospital patients. *Psychol Med* 1982; 12(2):397–408.

Archbold P. The impact of chronic illness in a parent on the middle-aged or elderly caregiver. Paper presented at the 31st Annual Meeting of the Gerontological Society of America, Dallas, TX, 1978.

Arnsten AFT, Goldman-Rakic PS. Alpha 2-adrenergic mechanisms in prefrontal cortex associated with cognitive decline in aged nonhuman primates. *Science* 1985; 230(4731):1273–1276.

Aronson MK, Lipkowitz R. Senile dementia, Alzheimer's type: The family and the health care delivery system. *J Am Geriatr Soc* 1981; 29(12):568–571.

Ashford JW, Ford CV. Use of MAO inhibitors in elderly patients. *Am J Pyschiatry* 1979; 136(11):1466–1467.

Ayres S Jr, Mihan R. Nocturnal leg cramps (systremma): A progress report on response to Vitamin E. *South Med J* 1974; 67(11):1308–1312.

Baker N. Reminiscing in group therapy for self-worth. *Journal of Gerontological Nursing* 1985; 11(7):21–24.

Barbeau A, Growdon JH, Wurtman RJ (eds.). *Nutrition and the Brain*, Vol. 5. New York: Raven Press, 1979.

Barclay LL, Zemcov A, Blass JP, Sansone J. Survival in Alzheimer's disease and vascular dementias. *Neurology* 1985; 35(6):834–840.

Barnes R, Raskind MA, Scott M, Murphy C. Problems of families caring for Alzheimer patients: Use of a support group. *J Am Geriatr Soc* 1981; 29(2):80–85.

Barnes R, Veith R, Okimoto J, Raskind M, Gumbrecht G. Efficacy of antipsychotic medications in behaviorally disturbed dementia patients. *Am J Psychiatry* 1982; 139(9):1170–1174.

Bartol MA. Dialogue with dementia. *Journal of Gerontological Nursing* 1979; 5(4):21–31.

Barton R, Hurst, L. Unnecessary use of tranquilizers in elderly patients. *Br J Psychiatry* 1966; 112:989–990.

Bartus RT, Dean RL III, Sherman KA, Friedman E, Beer B. Profound effects of combining choline and piracetam on memory enhancement and cholinergic function in aged rats. *Neurobiol Aging* 1981; 2(2):105–111.

Bartus RT, Dean RL III, Beer B, Lippa AS. The cholinergic hypothesis of geriatric memory dysfunction. *Science* 1982; 217(4558):408–417.

Beam IM. Helping families survive. *Am J Nurs* 1984; 84(2):228–232.

Beber CR. Management of behavior in the institutionalized aged. *Diseases of the Nervous System* 1965; 26:591–595.

Beck AT, Ward CH, Mendelson M, Mock J, Erbaugh J. An inventory for measuring depression. *Arch Gen Psychiatry* 1961; 4:561–571.

Behrendt JE. Alzheimer's disease and its effect on handwriting. *J Forensic Sci* 29(11):87–91, 1984.

Berg L. Mild senile dementia of the Alzheimer type: Diagnostic criteria and natural history. In TS Elizan (ed.), Alzheimer's and Parkinson's Diseases and the Aging Brain. *Mt Sinai J Med* 1988; 55(1).

Bergmann K, Foster EM, Justice AW, Matthews V. Management of the demented elderly patient in the community. *Br J Psychiatry* 1978; 132:441–449.

Berlin RM. Management of insomnia in hospitalized patients. *Ann Intern Med* 1984; 100(3):398–404.

Blass JP, Reding MJ, Drachman D, Mitchell A, Glosser G, Katzman R, Thal LJ, Grenell S, Spar JE, La Rue A. Cholinesterase inhibitors and opiate antagonists in patients with Alzheimer's disease [letter]. *N Engl J Med* 1983; 309(9):555–556.

Bliwise D, Carskadon M, Carey E, Dement W. Longitudinal development of sleep-related respiratory disturbance in adult humans. *J Gerontol* 1984; 39(3):290–293.

Bliwise D, Tinklenberg J, Davies H, Pursley A, Petta D, Yesavage J, Widrow L, Guilleminault C, Zarcone V, Dement WC. Sleep patterns in Alzheimer's disease. *Sleep Research* 1986; 15:49.

Bliwise DL, Feldman DE, Bliwise NG, Carskadon MA, Kraemer HC, North CS, Petta DF, Seidel WF, Dement WC. Risk factors for sleep disordered breath ing in heterogeneous geriatric populations. *J Am Geriatr Soc* 1987 35(2): 132–141.

Blowers AJ. Epidemiology of tardive dyskinesia in the elderly. *Neuropharmacology* 1981; 20(128):1339–1340.

Bondareff W, Mountjoy CQ, Roth M. Loss of neurons of origin of the adrenergic projection to cerebral cortex (nucleus locus ceruleus) in senile dementia. *Neurology* (NY) 1982; 32(2):164–168.

Borthwick NM, Yates CM, Gordon A. Reduced proteins in temporal cortex in Alzheimer's disease: An electrophoretic study. *J Neurochem* 1985; 44(5):1436–1441.

Bourgeois M, Bouilh P, Tignol J, Yesavage J. Spontaneous dyskinesias vs. neuroleptic-induced dyskinesias in 270 elderly subjects. *J Nerv Ment Dis* 1980; 168(3):177–178.

Bowen DM, Smith CB, White P, Davison AN. Neurotransmitter related enzymes and indices of hypoxia in senile dementia and other abiotrophies. *Brain* 1976; 99(3):459–496.

Bradshaw JR, Thomson JLG, Campbell MJ. Computed tomography in the investigation of dementia [clin res]. *Br Med J* 1983; 286(6361):277–280.

Branconnier RJ, Cole JO. The therapeutic role of methylphenidate in senile organic brain syndrome. In Cole JO, Barrett JE (Eds.), *Psychopathology in the Aged*. New York: Raven Press, 1980, pp. 183.–196.

Branconnier RJ, Cole JO, Ghazvinian S. The therapeutic profile of mianserin in mild elderly depressives [proceedings]. *Psychopharmacol Bull* 1981a; 17(1):129–131.

Branconnier RJ, DeVitt D, Cole JO. Evaluation of drug efficacy in dementia: A computerized cognitive assessment system. *Psychopharmacol Bull* 1981b; 17(1):4–6.

Branconnier RJ. The efficacy of the cerebral metabolic enhancers in the treatment of senile dementia. *Psychopharmacol Bull* 1983; 19(2):212–219.

Breeze J. The care of the aged. *Am J Nurs* 1909; 9(11):826–831.

Breitner JC, Folstein MF. Familial Alzheimer dementia: A prevalent disorder with specific clinical features. *Psychol Med* 1984; 14(1):63–80.

Brezinova V, Oswald I. Sleep after a bedtime beverage. *Br Med J* 1972; 2:431–433.

Brinkman SD, Smith RC, Meyer JS, Vroulis G, Shaw T, Gordon JR, Allen RH. Lecithin and memory training in suspected Alzheimer's disease. *J Gerontol* 1982; 37(1):4–9.

Brocklehurst JC. *Incontinence in Old People*. Edinburgh: Livingstone, 1951, pp. 92–127.

Brocklehurst JC. Bowel management in the neurologically disabled. The problems of old age. *Proc Roy Soc Med* 1972; 65:66–69.

Brocklehurst JC, Kirkland JL, Martin J, Ashford J. Constipation in long-stay elderly patients: Its treatment and prevention by lactulose, poloxalkoldihydroxyanthroquinolone and phosphate enemas. *Gerontology* 1983; 29(3):181–184.

Brody EM, Gummer B. Aged applicants and non-applicants to a voluntary home: An exploratory comparison. *Gerontologist* 1967; 7(4):234–243.

Brody EM. Follow-up study of applicants and non-applicants to a voluntary home. *Gerontologist* 1969; 9(3):187–196.

Brody EM, Kleban MH, Lawton MP, Silverman H. Excess disabilities of mentally impaired aged: Impact of individualized treatment. *Gerontologist* 1971; 11(2):124–133.

Brody EM. *Long-term Care of Older People: A Practical Guide.* New York: Human Sciences Press, 1977.

Brody EM. The aging of the family. *The Annals of the American Academy of Political and Social Science* 1978; 438:13–27.

Brody EM. The formal support network: Congregate treatment settings for residents with senescent brain dysfunction. In GD Cohen and NE Miller (eds.), *Clinical Aspects of Alzheimer's Disease and Senile Dementia*, Vol 15: *Aging.* New York: Raven Press, 1981a, pp. 301–331.

Brody EM. 'Women in the middle' and family help to older people. *Gerontologist* 1981b; 21(5):471–480.

Brody EM, Johnsen PT, Fulcomer MC, Lang AM. Women's changing roles and help to elderly parents: Attitudes of three generations of women. *J Gerontol* 1983; 38(5):597–607.

Brody EM, Lawton MP, Liebowitz B. Senile dementia: Public policy and adequate institutional care. *Am J Public Health* 1984a; 74(12):1381–1383.

Brody EM, Kleban MH, Johnsen PT. Women who provide parent care: Those who work and those who do not. Paper presented at the 37th annual meeting of the Gerontological Society of America. San Antonio, TX, 1984b.

Brody EM. *Mental and Physical Health Practices of Older People: A Guide for Health Professionals.* New York: Springer Publishing Co., 1985a.

Brody EM. Parent care as a normative family stress. *Gerontologist* 1985b; 25(1):19–29.

Brody EM, Schoonover C. Patterns of parent care when adult daughters work and when they do not. *Gerontologist* 1986; 26(4):372–381.

Brody EM, Kleban MH, Johnsen PT, Hoffman C, Schoonover C. Work status and parent care: A comparison of four groups of women. *Gerontologist* 1987; 27(2):201–208.

Brody EM. Filial care of the elderly and changing roles of women (and men). *J Geriatr Psychiatry* (in press).

Brody SJ, Poulshock SW, Masciocchi CF. The family caring unit: A major consideration in the long-term support system. *Gerontologist* 1978; 18(6):556–561.

Brody SJ. The thirty-to-one paradox: Health needs and medical solutions. In JP Hubbard (ed.), *Aging: Agenda for the Eighties, National Journal Issues Book.* Washington, DC: The Government Research Corporation, 1979, pp. 17–20.

Brown P. An epidemiologic critique of Creutzfeldt-Jakob disease. *Epidemiol Rev* 1980; 2:113–135.

Buchner DM, Larson EB. Is morbidity due to falls preventable in patients with dementia? *Clin Res* 1986; 34(2):810a.

Burnside IM. Alzheimer's disease: An overview. *Journal of Gerontological Nursing* 1979; 5(4):14–20.

Burnside IM, Moehrlin BA. Health care of the confused elderly at home. In S Ryan, C Wassenberg (eds.), *Nurs Clin North Am*, Vol. 15(2). Philadelphia: WB Saunders, 1980, pp. 389–402.

Burnside IM. Interviewing the confused aged person. In IM Burnside (ed.), *Psychosocial Nursing Care of the Aged*, 2nd ed. New York: McGraw-Hill, 1980a, pp. 19–33.

Burnside IM. Wandering behavior. In IM Burnside (ed.), *Psychosocial Nursing Care of the Aged*, 2nd ed. New York: McGraw-Hill, 1980b, pp. 298–309.

Burnside IM. Organic brain syndrome: Theory and therapy. In IM Burnside (ed.),

Nursing and the Aged, 2nd ed. New York: McGraw-Hill, 1981, pp. 167–200.

Burnside IM. The Alzheimer's disease patient in the nursing home. *Extension* 1982a; 2(4):1–2.

Burnside IM. Care of the Alzheimer patient in an institution. *Generations* 1982b; 7(1):22–24.

Burnside IM. Group work with the cognitively impaired. In IM Burnside (ed.), *Working with the Elderly: Group Process and Techniques,* 2nd ed. Monterey, CA: Jones & Bartlett, 1984, pp. 141–162.

Burnside IM, Baumler J, Weaver-Dyck S. Group work in a day care center. In IM Burnside (Ed.), *Working with the Elderly: Group Process and Techniques,* 2nd ed. Monterey, CA: Jones & Bartlett, 1984, pp. 78–88.

Burnside IM. Reminiscence therapy groups. *Extension* 1985; 5(3):2–4.

Buschke H, Fuld PA. Evaluating storage, retention, and retrieval in disorderd memory and learning. *Neurology* 1974; 24(11):1019–1025.

Caine ED. Pseudodementia. Current concepts and future directions. *Arch Gen Psychiatry* 1981; 38(12):1359–1364.

Caltagirone C, Gainotti G, Masullo C. Oral administration of chronic physostigmine does not improve cognitive or mnesic performances in Alzheimer's presenile dementia. *Int J Neurosci* 1982; 16(3–4):247–249.

Cameron DE. Studies in senile nocturnal delirium. *Psychiatr Q* 1941; 15(1):47–53.

Candy JM, Perry RH, Perry EK, Irving D, Blessed G, Fairbairn AF, Tomlinson BE. Pathological changes in the nucleus of Meynert in Alzheimer's and Parkinson's diseases. *J Neurol Sci* 1983; 59(2):277–289.

Candy JM, Klinowski J, Perry RH, Perry EK, Fairbairn AF, Oakley AE, Carpenter TA, Atack JR, Blessed G, Edwardson JA. Aluminosilicates and senile plaque formation in Alzheimer's disease. *Lancet* 1986; 1(8477):354–357.

Cantor MH. Neighbors and friends: An overlooked resource in the informal support system. *Res Aging* 1979; 1(4):434–463.

Cantor MH. Strain among caregivers: A study of experience in the United States. *Gerontologist* 1983; 23(6):597–604.

Carlisle EM, Curran MJ. Effect of dietary silicon and aluminum on silicon and aluminum levels in rat brain. *Alzheimer Disease and Associated Disorders* 1987; 1(2):83–89.

Carp RI, Merz GS, Wisniewski H. Transmission of unconventional slow virus diseases and the relevance to AD/SDAT transmission studies. In J Wertheimer, M Marois (eds.), *Senile Dementia: Outlook for the Future.* New York: Alan R. Liss, Inc., 1984, pp. 31–54.

Cassel CK, Jameton AL. Dementia in the elderly: An analysis of medical responsibility. *Ann Intern Med* 1981; 94(6):802–807.

Cerulli MA, Nikoomanesh P, Schuster MM. Progress in biofeedback conditioning for fecal incontinence. *Gastroenterology* 1979; 76(4):742–746.

Chapman LJ, Chapman JP. The measurement of differential deficit. *J Psychiatr Res* 1978; 14(1–4):303–311.

Cheah KC, Beard OW. Psychiatric findings in the population of a geriatric evaluation unit: Implications. *J Am Geriatr Soc* 1980; 28(4):153–156.

Chesrow EJ, Kaplitz SE, Vetra N, Breme JT, Marquardt GH. Double-blind study of oxazepam in the management of geriatric patients with behavioral problems. *Clinical Medicine* 1965; 72:1001–1005.

Christie JE, Shering A, Ferguson J, Glen AI. Physostigmine and arecoline: Effects of intravenous infusions in Alzheimer presenile dementia. *Br J Psychiatry* 1981; 138:46–50.

Coblentz JM, Mattis S, Zingesser LH, Kasoff SS, Wisniewski HM, Katzman R. Presenile dementia: Clinical aspects and evaluation of cerebrospinal fluid dynamics. *Arch Neurol* 1973; 29(5)299–308.

Cohen GD. Alzheimer's disease—the human concept. In R Katzman (ed.), *Biological Aspects of Alzheimer's Disease.* Banbury Report 15. Cold Spring Harbor, NY: Cold Spring Harbor Laboratory, 1983, pp. 3–6.

Cole JO. Drug therapy of senile organic brain syndromes. *Psychiatr J Univ Ottawa* 1980; 5:41–52.

Cole JO, Barrett JE (eds.). *Psychopathology in the Aged.* New York: Raven Press, 1980.

Cole JO, Branconnier RJ, Salomon M, Dessain E. Tricyclic use in the cognitively impaired elderly. *J Clin Psychiatry* 1983; 44(9, Pt 2):14–19.

Coleman RM, Miles LE, Guilleminault CC, Zarcone VP Jr, van den Hoed J, Dement WC. Sleep-wake disorders in the elderly: A polysomnographic analysis. *J Am Geriatr Soc* 1981; 29(7):289–296.

College Committee on Geriatrics. Organic mental impairment in the elderly. Implications for research, education and the provision of services. A report of the Royal College of Physicians. *J R Coll Physicians Lond* 1981; 15(3):141–167.

Comptroller General of the United States. *Home Health: The Need for a National Policy to Better Provide for the Elderly.* (HRD-78-19). Washington, DC: U.S. General Accounting Office, 1977a.

Comptroller General of the United States. *The Well-Being of Older People in Cleveland, Ohio.* (HRD-77-70). Washington, DC: U.S. General Accounting Office, 1977b.

Congress of the United States, Office of Technology Assessment. *Technology and Aging in America.* (OTA-BA-264). Washington, DC: U.S. Government Printing Office, 1985.

In re Claire C. Conroy, Supreme Court of New Jersey 98, N.J. 321, 486 A.2d 1209, January 17, 1985.

Cook P, James I. Cerebral vasodilators (first of two parts). *N Engl J Med* 1981; 305(25):1508–1513.

Corsellis JAN. Post-traumatic dementia. In R Katzman, RD Terry, KL Bick (eds.), *Alzheimer's Disease: Senile Dementia and Related Disorders,* Vol 7: *Aging.* New York: Raven Press, 1978, pp. 125–133.

Covington JS. Alleviating agitation, apprehension, and related symptoms in geriatric patients: A double-blind comparision of a phenothiazine and a benzodiazepine. *South Med J* 1975; 68(6):719–724.

Cox KG. Milieu therapy. *Geriatric Nursing* 1985; 6(3):152–154.

Creasey H, Rapoport SI. The aging human brain. *Ann Neurol* 1985; 17(1):2–10.

Crook T, Gershon S (eds.). *Strategies for the Development of an Effective Treatment for Senile Dementia.* New Canaan, CT: Mark Powley Associates, Inc., 1981.

Crook T. Clinical drug trials in Alzheimer's disease. *Ann NY Acad Sci* 1985; 444:428–436.

Danis BG. Stress in individuals caring for ill elderly relatives. Paper presented at the 31st annual meeting of the Gerontological Society of America, Dallas, TX, 1978.

Danish Medical Association. *Dan Med Bull* 1985; 32(Suppl 1):1–111.

Davies P, Maloney AJ. Selective loss of central cholinergic neurons in Alzheimer's disease [letter]. *Lancet* 1976; 2(8000):1403.

Davies P, Verth AH. Regional distribution of muscarinic acetylcholine receptor in normal and Alzheimer's-type dementia brains. *Brain Res* 1977; 138(2):385–392.

Davis CK. Statement before House Select Committee on Aging. In *Twentieth Anniversary of Medicare and Medicaid: Americans Still at Risk.* Washington, DC: U.S. Government Printing Office, July 30, 1985, pp. 20–34.

Delabar J-M, Goldgaber D, Lamour Y, Nicole A, Huret J-L, De Grouchy J, Brown P, Gajdusek DC, Sinet P-M. Beta amyloid gene duplication in Alzheimer's disease and karyotypically normal Down syndrome. *Science* 1987; 235(4794):1390–1392.

Delwaide PJ, Desseilles M. Spontaneous buccolinguofacial dyskinesia in the elderly. *Acta Neurol Scand* 1977; 56(3):256–262.

Demuth GW, Rand BS. Atypical major depression in a patient with severe primary degenerative dementia. *Am J Psychiatry* 1980; 137(12):1609–1610.

Denny-Brown D, Robertson EG. Investigation of nervous control of defaecation. *Brain* 1935; 58:256–310.

Dickinson VA. Maintenance of anal continence: A review of pelvic floor physiology. *Gut* 1978; 19(12):1163–1174.

Diesfeldt HFA, Diesfeldt-Groenendijk H. Improving cognitive performance in psychogeriatric patients: The influence of physical exercise. *Age Aging* 1977; 6(1):58–64.

DiFabio S. Nurses' reactions to restraining patients. *Am J Nurs* 1981; 81(5):973–975.

Dodd KJ, Holden A, Reed C. A census of elderly people in care. *Social Work Today* 1979; 10(46):10–14.

Doty P, Liu K, Wiener J. An overview of long-term care. *Health Care Financing Review* 1985; 6(3):69–78.

Drachman DA, Leavitt J. Human memory and the cholinergic system. *Arch Neurol* 1974; 30(2):113–121.

Drugs that cause psychiatric symptoms. In M Abramowicz (ed.), *The Medical Letter on Drugs and Therapeutics* 1986; 28(721):81–86.

Dunning WF, Curtis MR, Maun ME. The effect of added dietary tryptophane on the occurrence of 2-acetylaminofluorene-induced liver and bladder cancer in rats. *Cancer Res* 1950; 10:454–459.

Duthie HL, Gairns FW. Sensory nerve endings and sensation in the anal region of man. *Br J Surg* 1960; 47(206):585–595.

Eckholm E. New programs sought for caretakers of the aged. *The New York Times,* July 13, 1985, p. 44.

Edelson J, Lyons W. *Institutional Care of the Mentally Impaired Elderly.* New York: Van Nostrand Reinhold, Co., Inc., 1985.

Edwards H. The significance of brain damage in persistent oral dyskinesia. *Br J Psychiatry* 1970; 116:271–275.

Eggert GM, Brodows BS. The ACCESS program: Assuring quality in long-term care. *QRB* 1982; 8(2):10–15.

Eisdorfer C, Cohen D, Preston C. Behavioral and psychological therapies for the older patient with cognitive impairment. In NE Miller, GD Cohen (eds.),

Clinical Aspects of Alzheimer's Disease and Senile Dementia, Vol 15: *Aging.* New York: Raven Press, 1981, pp. 209–226.

Eisdorfer C, Cohen D. Management of the patient and family coping with dementing illness. *J Fam Pract* 1981; 12(5):831– 837.

Eliopoulos C. A self-care model for gerontological nursing. *Geriatric Nursing* 1984; 5(8):366–369.

Erickson R. Companion animals and the elderly. *Geriatric Nursing* 1985; 6(2):92–96.

Evans L. Sundown syndrome in the elderly: A phenomenon in search of exploration. *Center for the Study of Aging Newsletter* 1985; 7(3):7.

Facts and Comparisons: A Loose-leaf Drug Information Service. St. Louis: J.B. Lippincott, 1987.

Faden R, Beauchamp T. *A History and Theory of Informed Consent.* New York: Oxford University Press, 1986.

Fengler AP, Goodrich N. Wives of elderly disabled men: The hidden patients. *Gerontologist* 1979; 19(2):175–183.

Ferris SH, Sathananthan G, Reisberg B, Gershon S. Long-term choline treatment of memory-impaired elderly patients. *Science* 1979; 205(4410):1039–1040.

Ferris SH: Empirical studies in senile dementia with central nervous system stimulants and metabolic enhancers. In T Crook & S Gershon (eds.), *Strategies for the Development of an Effective Treatment for Senile Dementia.* New Canaan, CT: Mark Powley Associates, Inc., 1981, pp. 173–187.

Fitten LJ, Hamann C, Evans G, Kelley F, Smith E. Assessment of treatment and decision making competence in nursing home residents [abstract]. *J Am Geriatr Soc* 1984; 32(4)(Suppl 19).

Folstein MF, Folstein SE, McHugh PR. 'Mini-mental state.' A practical method for grading the cognitive state of patients for the clinician. *J Psychiatr Res* 1975; 12(3):189–198.

Folstein M, Powell D, Breitner J. The cognitive pattern of familial Alzheimer's disease. In R Katzman (ed.), *Biological Aspects of Alzheimer's Disease.* Banbury Report 15. Cold Spring Harbor, NY: Cold Spring Harbor Laboratory, 1983, pp. 337–349.

Fontaine L, Grand M, Chabert J, Szarvasi E, Bayssat M. Pharmacologie generale d'une substance nouvelle vasodilatrice, le naftridrofuryl. [Pharmacology of naftridrofuryl, a new vasodilatory.] *Chimica Therapeutica* 1968; 3(6):463–469.

Fozard JL. Normal and pathological age differences in memory. In JC Brocklehurst (ed.), *Textbook of Geriatric Medicine and Gerontology,* 3rd ed. Edinburgh, Scotland: Churchill Livingstone, 1985, pp. 122–144.

Frankfather D, Smith MJ, Caro FG. *Family Care of the Elderly: Public Initiatives and Private Obligations.* Lexington, MA: Heath, 1981.

Frommlet M, Prinz P, Vitiello MV, Ries R, Williams D. Sleep hypoxemia and apnea are elevated in females with mild Alzheimer's disease. *Sleep Research* 1986; 15:189.

Fu TK, Matsuyama SS, Kessler JO, Jarvik LF. Philothermal response, microtubules and dementia. *Neurobiol Aging* 1986; 7:41–43.

Fuller J, Ward E, Evans A, Massam K, Gardner A. Dementia: Supportive groups for relatives. *Br Med J* 1979; 1(6179):1684–1685.

Gallagher DE. Intervention strategies to assist caregivers of frail elderly: Current research status and future research directions. In C Eisdorfer, MP Lawton, & GL Maddox (eds.), *Annual Review of Gerontology and Geriatrics,* Vol 5. New York: Springer Publishing Co., 1985, pp. 249–282.

Gallagher D, Wrabetz A, Lovett S, Del Maestro S, Rose J. Depression and other negative affects in family caregivers. In E Light & B Lebowitz (eds.), *Alzheimer's Disease Treatment and Family Stress: Directions for Research*. Washington, DC: National Institute of Mental Health (in press).

Geddes JW, Monaghan DT, Cotman CW, Lott IT, Kim RC, Chui HC. Plasticity of hippocampal circuitry in Alzheimer's disease. *Science* 1985; 230(4730):1179–1181.

George LK. *Caregiver Well-Being: Correlates and Relationships with Participation in Community and Self-Help Groups*. Final report submitted to the AARP Andrus Foundation; Washington, DC: 1983.

George LK. *The Dynamics of Caregiver Burden*. Final report submitted to the AARP Andrus Foundation; 1984.

Georgotas A, Friedman E, McCarthy M, Mann J, Krakowski M, Siegel R, Ferris S. Resistant geriatric depressions and therapeutic response to monoamine oxidase inhibitors. *Biol Psychiatry* 1983; 18(2):195–205.

Gerner R, Estabrook W, Steuer J, Jarvik L. Treatment of geriatric depression with trazodone, imipramine and placebo: A double-blind study. *J Clin Psychiatry* 1980; 41(6):216–220.

Gibson GE, Shimada M, Blass JP. Alterations in acetylcholine synthesis and cyclic nucleotides in mild cerebral hypoxia. *J Neurochem* 1978; 31(4):757–760.

Gibson MJ. An international update on family care for the ill elderly. *Ageing International* 1982; 9(1):11–14.

Gibson MJ. Women and aging. Paper presented at International Symposium on Aging, Georgian Court College, Lakewood, NJ, October 1984.

Giurgea C. Nootropic and related drugs interacting with the integrative activity of the brain. In J Obiols, C Ballus, C Gonzalez-Monclus, & J Pujol (eds.), *Biological Psychiatry Today*. Amsterdam: Elsevier/North Holland Biomedical Press, 1979, pp. 876–881.

Gobert JG. Genèse d'un médicament: Le Piracetam metabolisation et recherche biochimique. [Development of a drug: The biochemistry and metabolism of piracetam.] *J Pharm Belg* 1972; 26:281–304.

Goldberg RJ. Care of demented elderly persons [letter]. *Ann Intern Med* 1981; 95(6):781.

Goldgaber D, Lerman MI, McBride OW, Saffiotti U, Gajdusek DC. Characterization and chromosomal localization of a cDNA encoding brain amyloid of Alzheimer's disease. *Science* 1987; 235(4791):877–880.

Goldman HH, Cohen GD, Davis M. Expanded Medicare outpatient coverage for Alzheimer's disease and related disorders [clinical conference]. *Hosp Community Psychiatry* 1985; 36(9):939–942.

Goldstein K. Function disturbances in brain damage. In S Arieti (ed.), *American Handbook of Psychiatry*, Vol 1. New York: Basic Books, Inc., 1969, pp. 770–794.

Goodnick P, Gershon S. Chemotherapy of cognitive disorders in geriatric subjects. *J Clin Psychiatry* 1984; 45(5):196–209.

Gootnick A. Night cramps and quinine. *Arch Intern Med* 1943; 71:555–562.

Gottfries CG, Adolfsson R, Aquilonius SM, Carlson A, Eckernas SA, Nordberg A, Oreland L, Svennerholm L, Wiberg A, Winblad B. Biochemical changes in dementia disorders of Alzheimer's type (AD/SDAT). *Neurobiol Aging* 1983; 4(4):261–271.

Greengold BA, Ouslander JG. Bladder retraining program for elderly patients with post-indwelling catheterization. *Journal of Gerontological Nursing* 1986; 12(6):31–35.

Growdon JH. Clinical profiles of Alzheimer's disease. In CG Gottfries (ed.), *Normal Aging, Alzheimer's Disease and Senile Dementia: Aspects on Etiology, Pathogenesis, Diagnosis, and Treatment*. Brussels: Éditions de l'Université de Bruxelles, 1985, pp. 213–218.

Grundke-Iqbal I, Iqbal K, Quinan M, Tung YC, Zaidi MS, Wisniewski HM. Microtubule-associated protein tau: A component of Alzheimer paired helical filaments. *J Biol Chem* 1986; 261:6084–6089.

Grunhaus L, Dilsaver S, Greden JF, Carroll BJ. Depressive pseudodementia: A suggested diagnostic profile. *Biol Psychiatry* 1983; 18(2):215–225.

Guilleminault C, Silvestri R. Aging, drugs and sleep. *Neurobiol Aging* 1982; 3(4):379–386.

Gurland B, Dean L, Gurland R, Cook D. Personal time dependency in the elderly of New York City: Findings from the U.S.–U.K. cross national geriatric community study. In *Dependency in the Elderly of New York City*. [Report of a Research Utilization Workshop held on March 23, 1978.] New York: Community Council of Greater New York, 1978, pp. 9–45.

Gurland BJ. The borderlands of dementia: The influence of sociocultural characteristics on rates of dementia occurring in the senium. In NE Miller, GD Cohen (eds.), *Clinical Aspects of Alzheimer's Disease and Senile Dementia*, Vol 15: *Aging*. New York: Raven Press, 1981, pp. 61–84.

Hachinski VC, Iliff LD, Zilhka E, DuBoulay GH, McAllister VL, Marshall J, Russell RW, Symon L. Cerebral blood flow in dementia. *Arch Neurol* 1975; 32(9):632–637.

Hagnell O, Lanke J, Rorsman B, Ojesjo L. Does the incidence of age psychosis decrease? A prospective, longitudinal study of a complete population investigated during the 25-year period 1947–1972: The Lundby study. *Neuropsychobiology* 1981; 7(4):201–211.

Hall BA. Toward an understanding of stability in nursing phenomena. *Advances in Nursing Science* 1983; 5(3):15–20.

Hamilton M. A rating scale for depression. *J Neurol Neurosurg Psychiatry* 1960; 23(1):56–62.

Hamilton LD, Bennett JL. Acetophenazine for hyperactive geriatric patients. *Geriatrics* 1962a; 17:596–601.

Hamilton LD, Bennett JL. The use of trifluoperazine in geriatric patients with chronic brain syndrome. *J Am Geriatr Soc* 1962b; 10:140–147.

Harbaugh RE, Roberts DW, Coombs DW, Saunders RL, Reeder TM. Preliminary report: Intracranial cholinergic drug infusion in patients with Alzheimer's disease. *Neurosurgery* 1984; 15(4):514–518.

Hartmann E. L tryptophan: A rational hypnotic with clinical potential. *Am J Psychiatry* 1977; 134(4):366–370.

Hartmann E, Lindsley JG, Spinweber C. Chronic insomnia: Effects of tryptophan, flurazepam, secobarbital and placebo. *Psychopharmacology* (Berlin) 1983; 80(2):138–142.

Havens WW 2d, Cole JO. Successful treatment of dementia with lithium [letter]. *J Clin Psychopharmacol* 1982; 2(1):71–72.

Hayter J. Patients who have Alzheimer's disease. *Am J Nurs* 1974; 74(8):1460–1463.

Heston LL. Dementia of the Alzheimer type: A perspective from family studies. In R Katzman (ed.), *Biological Aspects of Alzheimer's Disease*. Banbury Report 15. Cold Spring Harbor, NY: Cold Spring Harbor Laboratory, 1983, pp. 183–191.

Heyman A, Wilkinson WE, Hurwitz BJ, Schmechel D, Sigmon AH, Weinberg T,

Helms MJ, Swift M. Alzheimer's disease: Genetic aspects and associated clinical disorders. *Ann Neurol* 1983; 14(5):507–515.

Hicks R, Dysken MW, Davis JM, Lesser J, Ripeckyj A, Lazarus L. The pharmacokinetics of psychotropic medication in the elderly: A review. *J Clin Psychiatry* 1981; 42(10):374–385.

Himmelhoch JM, Neil JF, May SJ, Fuchs CZ, Licata SM. Age, dementia, dyskinesias and lithium response. *Am J Psychiatry* 1980; 137(8):941–945.

Hirschfeld MJ. Self-care potential: Is it present? *Journal of Gerontological Nursing* 1985; 11(8):28–34.

Hoenig J, Hamilton MW. Elderly psychiatric patients and the burden on the household. *Psychiatria et Neurologia* 1966; 152(5):281–293.

Hoffman C, Brody EM, Kleban MH. Parent care and depression: Differences between working and nonworking adult daughters. Paper presented at the 37th annual meeting of the Gerontological Society of America, San Antonio, TX, 1984.

Hollister LE, Yesavage J. Ergoloid mesylates for senile dementias: Unanswered questions. *Ann Intern Med* 1984; 100(6):894–898.

Holman BL, Gibson RE, Hill TC, Eckelman WC, Albert M, Reba RC. Muscarinic acetylcholine receptors in Alzheimer's disease: In vivo imaging with iodine 123-labeled 3-Quinuclidinyl-4-Iodobenzilate and emission tomography. *JAMA* 1985; 254(21):3063–3066.

Horl J, Rosenmayr L. Assistance to the elderly as a common task of the family and social service organization. *Arch Gerontol Geriatr* 1982; 1(1):75–95.

Horne JA. The effects of exercise upon sleep: A critical review. *Biol Psychol* 1981; 12(4):241–290.

Horowitz A. The role of families in providing long-term care to the frail and chronically ill elderly living in the community. Final report submitted to the Health Care Financing Administration, Department of Health and Human Services. Available as PB 84-135524, National Technical Information Service, Springfield, VA. May 1982.

Horowitz A, Dono JE, Brill R. Continuity or change in informal support? The impact of an expanded home care program. Paper presented at the 36th annual meeting of the Gerontological Society of America. San Francisco, 1983.

Horowitz A. Family caregiving to the frail elderly. In C Eisdorfer, MP Lawton, GL Maddox (eds.), *Annual Review of Gerontology and Geriatrics*, Vol. 5. New York: Springer Publishing Co., 1985a, pp. 194–246.

Horowitz A. Sons and daughters as caregivers to older parents: Differences in role performance and consequences. *Gerontologist* 1985b; 25(6):612–617.

House Select Committee on Aging. *Twentieth Anniversary of Medicare and Medicaid: Americans Still at Risk.* Washington, DC: U.S. Government Printing Office, July 30, 1985.

Hu T, Huang LF, Cartwright WS. Evaluation of costs of caring for the senile demented elderly: A pilot study. *Gerontologist* 1986; 26(2): 158–163.

Huang LF, Cargwright WS, Hu T. The economic cost of senile dementia in the United States. Manuscript to be published in *Public Health Reports*, U.S. Public Health Service, January-February, 1988.

Huey FL. What teaching nursing homes are teaching us. *Am J Nurs* 1985; 85(6):678–683.

Hughes JR, Williams JG, Currier RD. An ergot alkaloid preparation (Hydergine) in the treatment of dementia: Critical review of the clinical literature. *J Am Geriatr Soc* 1976; 24(11):490–497.

Hunt A. *The Elderly at Home*. Office of Population Censuses and Surveys. London: Her Majesty's Stationery Office, 1978.

Ihre T. Studies on anal function in continent and incontinent patients. *Scand J Gastroenterol* 1974; 9(Suppl 25):1–64.

Inglis J. A paired-associate learning test for use with elderly psychiatric patients. *Journal of Mental Science* 1959; 105(439):440–443.

International Classification of Diseases Clinical Modification, 9th rev. ed. Geneva: World Health Organization, 1980.

Iqbal K, Zaidi T, Wen GY, Grundke-Iqbal I, Merz PA, Shaikh SS, Wisniewski HM, Alafuzoff I, Winblad B. Defective brain microtubule assembly in Alzheimer's disease. *Lancet* 1986; 2(8504):421–426.

Ishii T. Distribution of Alzheimer's neurofibrillary changes in the brain stem and hypothalamus of senile dementia. *Acta Neuropathol* (Berlin) 1966; 6:181–187.

Itil TM, Reisberg B, Huque M, Mehta D. Clinical profiles of tardive dyskinesia. *Compr Psychiatry* 1981; 22(3):282–290.

Itil TM, Menon GN, Bozak M, Songar A. The effects of oxiracetam (ISF 2522) in patients with organic brain syndrome (a double-blind controlled study with piracetam). *Drug Development Research* 1982; 2(5):447–461.

Itil TM. Nootropics: Status and prospects. *Biol Psychiatry* 1983; 18(5):521–523.

Jarrett AS, Exton-Smith AN. Treatment of faecal incontinence [letter]. *Lancet* 1960; 1(7130):925.

Jarvik LF, Greenblatt DJ, Harman D (eds.). *Clinical Pharmacology and the Aged Patient*, Vol. 16: *Aging*. New York: Raven Press, 1981.

Jarvik LF, Matsuyama SS, Kessler JO, Fu TK, Tsai SY, Clark EO. Philothermal response of polymorphonuclear leukocytes in dementia of the Alzheimer type. *Neurobiol Aging* 1982; 3:93–99.

Jarvik LF. Age is in—Is the wit out? In D Samuel, S Algeri, S Gershon, VE Grimm, G Toffano (eds.), *Aging of the Brain*, Vol. 22: *Aging*. New York: Raven Press, 1983, pp. 1–8.

Jenike MA. Monoamine oxidase inhibitors as treatment for depressed patients with primary degenerative dementia (Alzheimer's disease). *Am J Psychiatry* 1985; 142(6):763–764.

Jervis GA. Early senile dementia in mongoloid idiocy. *Am J Psychiatry* 1948; 105:102–106.

Johns CA, Greenwald BS, Mohs RC, Davis KL. The cholinergic treatment strategy in aging senile dementia. *Psychopharmacol Bull* 1983; 19(2):185–197.

Johns CA, Haroutunian V, Greenwald BS, Mohs RC, Davis BM, Kanof P, Horvath TB, Davis KL. Development of cholinergic drugs for the treatment of Alzheimer's disease. *Drug Development Research* 1985; 5(1):77–96.

Johnson C. Impediments to family supports to dependent elderly. Paper presented at the 32nd annual scientific meeting of the Gerontological Society of America, Washington, DC, 1979.

Johnson CL, Catalano DJ. A longitudinal study of family supports to impaired elderly. *Gerontologist* 1983; 23(6):612–618.

Jones IH. Senile dementia. *Nursing Times* 1979; 75(3):104–106.

Jones MK. Patient violence. Report of 200 incidents. *J Psychosoc Nurs Ment Health Serv* 1985; 23(6):12–17.

Jonsen AR. *Clinical Ethics: A Practical Approach to Ethical Decisions in Clinical Medicine*. New York: Macmillan, 1982.

Jorm AF. Subtypes of Alzheimer's dementia: A conceptual analysis and critical review. *Psychol Med* 1985; 15(3):543–553.

Jotkowitz S. Lack of clinical efficacy of chronic oral physostigmine in Alzheimer's disease. *Ann Neurol* 1983; 14(6):690–691.

Kahn RL, Goldfarb AI, Pollack M, Peck A. Brief objective measures for the determination of mental status in the aged. *Am J Psychiatry* 1960; 117:326–328.

Kahn RL, Tobin SS. Community treatment for aged persons with altered brain function. In NE Miller & GD Cohen (eds.), *Clinical Aspects of Alzheimer's Disease and Senile Dementia,* Vol. 15: *Aging.* New York: Raven Press, 1981, pp. 253–276.

Kales A, Kales JD. Sleep disorders. Recent findings in the diagnosis and treatment of disturbed sleep. *N Engl J Med* 1974; 290:487–499.

Kales A, Bixler EO, Soldatos CR, Vela-Bueno A, Caldwell AB, Cadieux RJ. Biopsychobehavioral correlates of insomnia, Part 1: Role of sleep apnea and nocturnal myoclonus. *Psychosomatics* 1982; 23(6):589–600.

Kales A, Soldatos CR, Bixler EO, Kales JD. Early morning insomnia with rapidly eliminated benzodiazepines. *Science* 1983; 220(4592):95–97.

Kallmann FJ. *Heredity in Health and Mental Disorder.* New York: Norton, 1953.

Kang J, Lemaire H-G, Unterbeck A, Salbaum JM, Masters CL, Grzeschik K-H, Multhaup G, Beyreuther K, Muller-Hill B. The precursor of Alzheimer's disease amyloid A4 protein resembles a cell-surface receptor. *Nature* 1987; 325:733–736.

Katz S, Downs TD, Cash HR, Grotz RC. Progress in development of the index of ADL. *Gerontologist* 1970; 10(1):20–30.

Katzman R. Alzheimer's disease. *N Engl J Med* 1986; 314(15):964–973.

Kay DW, Beamish P, Roth M. Old age mental disorders in Newcastle-upon-Tyne. *Br J Psychiatry* 1964; 110:146–158.

Kay DW, Bergmann K, Foster EM, McKechnie AA, Roth M. Mental illness and hospital usage in the elderly: A random sample followed up. *Compr Psychiatry* 1970; 11(1):26–35.

Kaye WH, Sitaram N, Weingartner H, Ebert MH, Smallberg S, Gillin JC. Modest facilitation of memory in dementia with combined lecithin and anticholinesterase treatment. *Biol Psychiatry* 1982; 17(2):275–280.

Kegel A. Stress incontinence of urine in women: Physiologic treatment. *Journal of the International College of Surgeons* 1956; 25:487–499.

Kelwala S, Pomara N, Stanley M, Sitaram N, Gershon S. Lithium-induced accentuation of extrapyramidal symptoms in individuals with Alzheimer's disease. *J Clin Psychiatry* 1984; 45(8):342–344.

Kidd M, Allsop D, Landon M. Senile plaque amyloid, paired helical filaments, and cerebrovascular amyloid in Alzheimer's disease are all deposits of the same protein [letter]. *Lancet* 1985; 1(8423):278.

Kiloh LG. Pseudodementia. *Acta Psychiatr Scand* 1961; 37(4):336–351.

Kirshner HS, Webb WG, Kelly MP, Wells CE. Language disturbance: An initial symptom of cortical degenerations and dementia. *Arch Neurol* 1984; 41(5):491–496.

Kirven LE, Montero EF. Comparison of thioridazine and diazepam in the control of nonpsychotic symptoms associated with senility: Double-blind study. *J Am Geriatr Soc* 1973; 21:546–551.

Kitamoto T, Tateishi J, Tashima T, Takeshita I, Barry RA, DeArmond SJ, Prusiner SB. Amyloid plaques in Creutzfeldt-Jakob disease stain with prion protein antibodies. *Ann Neurol* 1986; 20:204–208.

Kleban MH, Brody EM, Lawton MP. Personality traits in the mentally impaired aged and their relationship to improvements in current functioning. *Gerontologist* 1971; 11(2):134–140.

Kroboth PD, Juhl RP. New drug evaluations: Triazolam. *Drug Intell Clin Pharm* 1983; 17(7–8):495–500.

Lang AM, Brody EM. Characteristics of middle-aged daughters and help to their elderly mothers. *Journal of Marriage and the Family* 1983; 45(1):193–202.

Lantz JM. In search of agents for self-care. *Journal of Gerontological Nursing* 1985; 11(7):10–14.

Larson EB, Reifler BV, Canfield C. Practical geriatrics: Evaluating elderly outpatients with symptoms of dementia. *Hosp Community Psychiatry* 1984; 35(5):425–428.

Larson EB, Reifler BV, Sumi SM, Canfield CG, Chinn NM. Diagnostic evaluation of 200 elderly outpatients with suspected dementia. *J Gerontol* 1985; 40(5):536–543.

Larson EB, Reifler BV, Sumi SM, Canfield CG, Chinn NM. Diagnostic tests in the evaluation of dementia: A prospective study of 200 elderly outpatients. *Arch Intern Med* 1986; 146(10):1917–1922.

Larson EB, Kukull WA, Buchner D, Reifler BV. Adverse drug reactions associated with global cognitive impairment in elderly persons. *Ann Intern Med* 1987; 107(2):169–173.

Larsson T, Sjogren T, Jacobson G. Senile dementia. A clinical, sociomedical and genetic study. *Acta Psychiatr Scand Suppl* 1963; 39(167):3–259.

La Rue A. Memory loss and aging. Distinguishing dementia from benign senescent forgetfulness and depressive pseudodementia. *Psychiatr Clin North Am* 1982; 5(1):89–103.

La Rue A, D'Elia LF, Clark EO, Spar JE, Jarvik LF. Clinical tests of memory in dementia, depression, and healthy aging. *Psychology and Aging* 1986a; 1(1):69–77.

La Rue A, Spar J, Dessonville Hill C. Cognitive impairment in late-life depression: Clinical correlates and treatment implications. *J Affective Disord* 1986b; 11:179–184.

Lawton MP, Brody EM: Assessment of older people: Self-maintaining and instrumental activities of daily living. *Gerontologist* 1969; 9(3):179–186.

Lawton MP, Moss M, Fulcomer M, Kleban MH. A research and service oriented multilevel assessment instrument. *J Gerontol* 1982; 37(1):91–99.

LeMay M. CT changes in dementing diseases: A review. *American Journal of Roentgenology* 1986; 147(5):963–975.

Levin HS, Peters BH. Long-term administration of oral physostigmine and lecithin improve memory in Alzheimer's disease [letter]. *Ann Neurol* 1984; 15(2):210.

Levy R, Little A, Chuaqui P, Reith M. Early results from double-blind, placebo controlled trial of high dose phosphatidylcholine in Alzheimer's disease [letter]. *Lancet* 1983; 1(8331):987–988.

Linnoila M, Viukari M. Efficacy and side effects of nitrazepam and thioridazine as sleeping aids in psychogeriatric inpatients. *Br J Psychiatry* 1976; 128:566–569.

Linnoila M, Viukari M, Numminen A, Auvinen J. Efficacy and side effects of chloral hydrate and tryptophan as sleeping aids in psychogeriatric patients. *International Pharmacopsychiatry* 1980; 15(2):124–128.

Lipowski ZJ. Transient cognitive disorders (delirium, acute confusional states) in the elderly. *Am J Psychiatry* 1983; 140(11):1426–1436.

Liston EH, Jarvik LF. Psychotherapy and pharmacotherapy in primary degenerative dementia. In NE Miller & GD Cohen (eds.), *Mental Health Aspects of Physical Disease in Late Life.* New York: Guilford Press (in press).

Little A, Levy R, Chuaqui-Kidd P, Hand D. A double-blind, placebo-controlled trial of high-dose lecithin in Alzheimer's disease. *J Neurol Neurosurg Psychiatry* 1985; 48(8):736–742.

Lynn J. Brief and appendix for amicus curiae: The American Geriatrics Society— In the matter of Claire C. Conroy. *J Am Geriatr Soc* 1984; 32(12):915–922.

Mace NL, Rabins PV. *The 36 Hour Day. A Family Guide to Caring for Persons with Alzheimer's Disease, Related Dementing Illness, and Memory Loss in Later Life.* Baltimore: Johns Hopkins University Press, 1982.

Mackey AM. OBS and nursing care. *Journal of Gerontological Nursing* 1983; 9(2):74–85.

Malech HL, Root RK, Gallin JI. Structural analysis of human neutrophil migration. Centriole, microtubule, and microfilament orientation and function during chemotaxis. *J Cell Biol* 1977; 75(3):666–693.

Mancillas JR, Siggins GR, Bloom FE. Systemic ethanol: Selective enhancement of responses to acetylcholine and somatostatin in hippocampus. *Science* 1986; 231(4734):161–163.

Martin JC, Ballinger BR, Cockram LL, McPherson FM, Pigache RM, Tregaskis D. Effect of a synthetic peptide, ORG 2766, on inpatients with severe senile dementia. A controlled clinical trial. *Acta Psychiatr Scand* 1983; 67(3):205–207.

Masters CL, Harris JO, Gajdusek DC, Gibbs CJ Jr, Bernoulli C, Asher DM. Creutzfeldt-Jakob disease: Patterns of worldwide occurrence and the significance of familial and sporadic clustering. *Ann Neurol* 1979; 5(2)177–188.

Masters CL, Gajdusek DC, Gibbs CJ Jr. The familial occurrence of Creutzfeldt-Jakob disease and Alzheimer's disease. *Brain* 1981; 104(3):535–558.

Matsuyama SS, Jarvik LF, Kumar V. Dementia: Genetics. In T Arie (ed.), *Recent Advances in Psychogeriatrics.* London: Churchill-Livingstone, 1985, pp. 45–69.

McAllister TW. Overview: Pseudodementia. *Am J Psychiatry* 1983; 140(5):528–533.

McAllister TW, Price TRP. Severe depressive pseudodementia with and without dementia. *Am J Psychiatry* 1983; 139(5):626–629.

McKhann G, Drachman D, Folstein M, Katzman R, Price D, Stadlan EM. Clinical diagnosis of Alzheimer's disease: Report of the NINCDS–ADRDA work group under the auspices of the Department of Health and Human Services Task Force on Alzheimer's disease. *Neurology* (NY) 1984; 34(7):939–944.

Meier-Ruge W, Enz A, Gygax P, Hunzikep O, Iwangoff P, Reichlmeier K. Experimental pathology in basic research of the aging brain. In S Gershon & A Raskin (eds.), *Genesis and Treatment of Psychologic Disorders in the Elderly,* Vol 2: *Aging.* New York: Raven Press, 1975, pp. 55–126.

Meltzer JW. *Respite Care: An Emerging Family Support Service.* Washington, DC: The Center for the Study of Social Policy, 1982.

Merritt TL. Equality for the elderly incompetent: A proposal for dignified death. *Stanford Law Review* 1987; 39(3):689–736.

Meyers BS, Mei-Tal V. Psychiatric reactions during tricyclic treatment of the elderly reconsidered. *J Clin Psychopharmacol* 1983; 3(1):2–6.

Meyers DW. Legal aspects of withdrawing nourishment from an incurably ill patient. *Arch Intern Med* 1985; 145(1):125–128.

Miles LE, Dement WB. Sleep and aging. *Sleep* 1980; 3(2):119–220.

Miller E. *Abnormal Aging: The Psychology of Senile and Presenile Dementia.* New York: Wiley, 1977.

Miller NE, Cohen GD (eds.). *Clinical Aspects of Alzheimer's Disease and Senile Dementia,* Vol 15: *Aging.* New York: Raven Press, 1981.

Miller RR, Greenblatt DJ. Clinical effects of chloral hydrate in hospitalized medical patients. *J Clin Pharmacol* 1979; 19(10):669–674.

Mizuki Y, Yamada M, Kato I, Takada Y, Tsujimaru S, Inanaga K, Tanaka M. Effects of aniracetam, a nootropic drug, in senile dementia—a preliminary report. *Kurume Medical Journal* 1984; 31(2):135–143.

Moehrlin B. Don't worry—she won't know. *Extension* 1985; 5(2):2–3.

Mohs RC, Davis KL. A signal detectability analysis of the effect of physostigmine on memory in patients with Alzheimer's disease. *Neurobiol Aging* 1982; 3(2):105–110.

Mohs RC, Rosen WG, Davis KL. Defining treatment efficacy in patients with Alzheimer's disease. In S Corkin, KL Davis, JH Growdon, E Usdin & RJ Wurtman (eds.), *Alzheimer's Disease: A Report of Progress in Research,* Vol 19: *Aging.* New York: Raven Press, 1982, pp. 351–356.

Mohs RC. Psychological tests for patients with moderate to severe dementia. In T Crook, S Ferris & R Bartus (eds.), *Assessment in Geriatric Psychopharmacology.* New Canaan, CT: Mark Powley Associates, Inc., 1983, pp. 169–176.

Mohs RC, Rosen WG, Greenwald BS, Davis KL. Neuropathologically validated scales for Alzheimer's disease. In T Crook, S Ferris, & R Bartus (eds.), *Assessment in Geriatric Psychopharmacology.* New Canaan, CT: Mark Powley Associates, Inc., 1983, pp. 37–45.

Mohs RC, Davis BM, Greenwald BS, Mathe AA, Johns CA, Horvath TB, Davis KL. Clinical studies of the cholinergic deficit in Alzheimer's disease: II. Psychopharmacologic studies. *J Am Geriatr Soc* 1985; 33(11):749–757.

Mortimer JA, Schuman LM, French LR. Epidemiology of dementing illness. In JA Mortimer & LM Schuman (eds.), *The Epidemiology of Dementia.* New York: Oxford University Press, 1981, pp. 3–23.

Mortimer JA, French LR, Hutton JT, Schuman LM. Head injury as a risk factor for Alzheimer's disease. *Neurology* 1985; 35(2):264–267.

Moss MS, Kurland P. Family visiting with institutionalized mentally impaired aged. *Journal of Gerontological Social Work* 1979; 1(4):271–278.

Mountjoy CQ, Roth M, Evans NJ, Evans HM. Cortical neuronal counts in normal elderly controls and demented patients. *Neurobiol Aging* 1983; 4(1):1–11.

Myllyluoma J, Soldo BJ. Family caregivers to the elderly: Who are they? Paper presented at the 33rd annual meeting of the Gerontological Society of America, San Diego, 1980.

National Center for Health Statistics. Advance Report of Final Natality Statistics, 1983. *Monthly Vital Statistics Report* (PHS-85-1120), Vol 34 (6)(Suppl). Hyattsville, MD: Public Health Service, September 20, 1985.

Naugle RI, Cullum CM, Bigler ED, Massman PJ. Neuropsychological and computerized axial tomography volume characteristics of empirically derived dementia subgroups. *J Nerv Ment Dis* 1985; 173(10):596–604.

Neshkes R, Gerner R, Jarvik LF, Mintz J, Joseph J, Linde S, Aldrich J, Conolly ME, Rosen R, Hill M. Orthostatic effects of imipramine and doxepin in depressed geriatric outpatients. *J Clin Psychopharmacol* 1985; 5(2):102–106.

New York City Department for the Aging. *Caring: A Family Guide To Managing the Alzheimer's Patient at Home.* New York: The New York City Alzheimer's Resource Center, 1985.

New York City Department for the Aging and The Brookdale Foundation. *Agendas for Action: The Aging Network Responds to Alzheimer's Disease.* New York: The New York City Alzheimer's Resource Center, 1986.

New York City Department for the Aging. *Alzheimer's Disease: Where To Go for Help in New York City,* 4th ed. New York: The New York City Alzheimer's Resource Center 1987.

New York State Health Advisory Council. Enhancing and sustaining informal support networks for the elderly and disabled: Recommendations to the New York State Health Advisory Council. Albany, NY: Health Planning Commission, 1981.

Niederehe G, Frugé E. Dementia and family dynamics: Clinical research issues. *J Geriatr Psychiatry* 1984; 17(1):21–60.

Nott PN, Fleminger JJ. Presenile dementia: The difficulties of early diagnosis. *Acta Psychiatr Scand* 1975; 51(3):210–217.

Nowakowski L. Accent capabilities in disorientation. *Journal of Gerontological Nursing* 1985; 11(9):15–20.

Obrist WD. Cerebral physiology of the aged. Influence of circulatory disorders. In CM Gaitz (ed.), *Aging and the Brain.* New York: Plenum Press, 1972, pp. 117–133.

Okawa KK. Comparison of triazolam 25mg and flurazepam 15mg in treating geriatric insomniacs. *Current Therapeutic Research* 1978; 23(3):381–387.

Olsen EJ, Bank L, Jarvik LF. Gerovital-H3: A clinical trial as an antidepressant. *J Gerontol* 1978; 33(4):514–520.

Orem DE. *Nursing: Concepts of Practice,* 3rd ed. New York: McGraw-Hill, 1985.

Ory MG, Williams TF, Emr M, Liebowitz B, Rabins P, Solloway J, Sluss-Raddaugh T, Wolff E, Zarit S. Families, informal supports, and Alzheimer's disease. *Res Aging* 1985; 7(4):623–643.

Ostfeld A, Smith CM, Stotsky BA. The systemic use of procaine in the treatment of the elderly: A review. *J Am Geriatr Soc* 1977; 25(1):1–19.

Pakes GE. L tryptophan in psychiatric practice. *Drug Intell Clin Pharm* 1979; 13(7–8):391–396.

Pakes GE, Brogden RN, Heel RC, Speight TM, Avery GS. Triazolam: A review of its pharmacological properties and therapeutic efficacy in patients with insomnia. *Drugs* 1981; 22(2):81–110.

Palmer MH. Alzheimer's disease and critical care: Interactions, implications, interventions. *Journal of Gerontological Nursing* 1983; 9(2):86–90.

Parks AG, Porter NH, Hardcastle JD. The syndrome of the descending perineum. *Proc Roy Soc Med* 1966; 59:477–482.

Parks AG, Swash M, Urich H. Sphincter denervation in anorectal incontinence and rectal prolapse. *Gut* 1977; 18(8):656–665.

Parks AG. Faecal incontinence. In D Mandelstam (ed.), *Incontinence and Its Management*. London: Croom Helm, 1980, pp. 76–93.

Patrick ML. Care of the confused elderly patient. *Am J Nurs* 1967; 67(12):2536–2539.

Peabody CA, Thiemann S, Pigache R, Miller TP, Berger PA, Yesavage J, Tinklenberg JR. Desglycinamide-9-arginine-8-vasopressin (DGAVP, Organon 5667) in patients with dementia. *Neurobiol Aging* 1985; 6(2):95–100.

Peck DA. Rectal mucosal replacement. *Ann Surg* 1980; 191(3):294–303.

Peppards NR. Alzheimer special-care nursing home units. *Nursing Homes* 1985; 34(5):25–28.

Percy JP, Neill ME, Kandiah TK, Swash M. A neurogenic factor in faecal incontinence in the elderly. *Age Ageing* 1982; 11(3):175–179.

Perry EK, Tomlinson BE, Blessed G, Bergmann K, Gibson PH, Perry RH. Correlation of cholinergic abnormalities with senile plaques and mental test scores in senile dementia. *Br Med J* 1978; 2(1650):1457–1459.

Perry EK, Perry RH. A review of neuropathological and neurochemical correlates of Alzheimer's disease. *Dan Med Bull* 1985; 32(Suppl 1):27–34.

Peters BH, Levin HS. Effects of physostigmine and lecithin on memory in Alzheimer's disease. *Ann Neurol* 1979; 6(3):219–221.

Petrie WM, Ban TA, Berney S, Fujimori M, Guy W, Ragheb M, Wilson WH, Schaffer JD. Loxapine in psychogeriatrics: A placebo- and standard-controlled clinical investigation. *J Clin Psychopharmacol* 1982; 2(2):122–126.

Pfeiffer E. A short portable mental status questionnaire for the assessment of organic brain deficit in elderly patients. *J Am Geriatr Soc* 1975; 23(10):433–441.

Phelps ME, Mazziotta JC. Positron emission tomography: Human brain function and biochemistry. *Science* 1985; 228(4701):799–809.

Physicians' Desk Reference, 41st ed. Oradell, NJ: Medical Economics Co., Inc., 1987.

Pinel C. Alzheimer's disease. *Nursing Times* 1975; 71(3):105–106.

Polk-Penrod E. The self-perceived needs of families caring for relatives with Alzheimer's disease. Unpublished master's thesis. Department of Nursing, San Jose State University, 1982.

Powter S. Senile dementia. *Nursing Mirror* 1977; 145(18):31–35.

President's Commission for the Study of Ethical Problems in Medicine and Biomedical and Behavioral Research. *Making Health Care Decisions, Vol. I: Report*. Washington DC: 1982.

Price JM. Bladder cancer. Canadian Cancer Conference 1966; 6:224–243.

Prien RF, Haber PA, Caffey EM Jr. The use of psychoactive drugs in elderly patients with psychiatric disorders: Survey conducted in twelve Veterans Administration hospitals. *J Am Geriatr Soc* 1975; 23(3):104–112.

Prinz PN, Peskind ER, Vitaliano PP, Raskind MA, Eisdorfer C, Zemcuznikov N, Gerber CJ. Changes in the sleep and waking EEGs of nondemented and demented elderly subjects. *J Am Geriatr Soc* 1982a; 30(2):86–93.

Prinz PN, Vitaliano PP, Vitiello MV, Bokan J, Raskind M, Peskind E, Gerber C. Sleep, EEG and mental function changes in senile dementia of the Alzheimer's type. *Neurobiol Aging* 1982b; 3:361–370.

Prinz PN, Frommlet M, Vitiello MV, Ries R, Williams D. Periodic leg movements are unaffected by mild Alzheimer's disease. *Sleep Research* 1986; 15:200.

Purtilo RB, Cassel CK. *Ethical Dimensions in the Health Professions*. Philadelphia: W. B. Saunders Co., 1981.

Quinn JB. Paying for a nursing home. *Newsweek*, June 24, 1985, p. 67.

Rabins PV, Mace NL, Lucas MJ. The impact of dementia on the family. *JAMA* 1982; 248(3):333–335.

Rada RT, Kellner R. Thiothixene in the treatment of geriatric patients with chronic organic brain syndrome. *J Am Geriatr Soc* 1976; 24(3):105–107.

Rader J, Doan J, Schwab M. How to decrease wandering: A form of agenda behavior. *Geriatric Nursing* 1985; 6(4):196–199.

Ramsey M. Providing a safe home environment. In C Browne & R Onzuka-Anderson (eds.), *Our Aging Parents: A Practical Guide to Eldercare*. Honolulu: University of Hawaii Press, 1985, pp. 176–185.

Rango N. The nursing home resident with dementia: Clinical care ethics and policy implications. *Ann Intern Med* 1985; 102(6):835–841.

Raskin A, Rae DS. Psychiatric symptoms in the elderly [proceedings]. *Psychopharmacol Bull* 1981; 17(1):96–99.

Raskin DE. Antipsychotic medication and the elderly. *J Clin Psychiatry* 1985; 46(5, Pt 2):36–40.

Reding MJ, DiPonte P. Vasopressin in Alzheimer's disease. *Neurology* 1983; 33(12):1634–1635.

Reeves RL. Comparison of triazolam, flurazepam and placebo as hypnotics in geriatric patients with insomnia. *J Clin Pharmacol* 1977; 17(5–6):319–323.

Regestein QR. Treatment of insomnia in the elderly. In C Salzman (ed.), *Clinical Geriatric Psychopharmacology*. New York: McGraw-Hill, Inc., 1984, pp. 149–170.

Reifler B, Eisdorfer C. A clinic for the impaired elderly and their families. *Am J Psychiatry* 1980; 137(11):1399–1403.

Reifler BV, Larsen E, Hanley R. Coexistence of cognitive impairment and depression in geriatric outpatients. *Am J Psychiatry* 1982; 139(5):623–626.

Reifler BV, Larson E, Teri L, Poulsen M. Dementia of the Alzheimer's type and depression. *J Am Geriatr Soc* 1986; 34(12):855–859.

Reisberg B. Empirical studies in senile dementia with metabolic enhancers and agents that alter blood flow and oxygen utilization. In T Crook & S Gershon (eds.), *Strategies for the Development of an Effective Treatment for Senile Dementia*. New Canaan, CT: Mark Powley Associates, Inc., 1981, pp. 189–206.

Reisberg B, Ferris SH. Diagnosis and assessment of the older patient. *Hosp Community Psychiatry* 1982; 33(2):104–110.

Reisberg B (ed.). *Alzheimer's Disease: The Standard Reference*. New York: The Free Press, 1983.

Reisberg B, Ferris SH, Anand R, Mir P, Geibel V, de Leon MJ, Roberts E. Effects of naloxone in senile dementia: A double-blind trial [letter]. *N Engl J Med* 1983a; 308(12):721–722.

Reisberg B, London E, Ferris SH, Anand R, de Leon MJ. Novel pharmacologic approaches to the treatment of senile dementia of the Alzheimer's type (SDAT). *Psychopharmacol Bull* 1983b; 19(2):220–225.

Reisberg B, Schneck MK, Ferris SH, Schwartz GE, de Leon MJ. The brief cognitive rating scale (BCRS): Findings in primary degenerative dementia (PDD). *Psychopharmacol Bull* 1983c; 19(1):47–50.

Reisberg B. Alzheimer's disease. Stages of cognitive decline. *Am J Nurs* 1984; 84(2):225–228.

Reisine TD, Yamamura HI, Bird ED, Spokes E, Enna SJ. Pre- and post-synaptic neurochemical alterations in Alzheimer's disease. *Brain Res* 1978; 159(2):477–481.

Reitan RM, Davison LA. *Clinical Neuropsychology: Current Status and Applications.* New York: Wiley, 1974.

Resnick NM. Urinary incontinence in the elderly. *Medical Grand Rounds* 1984; 3(3):281–290.

Reynolds CF 3d, Kupfer DJ, Taska LS, Hoch CC, Sewitch DE, Restifo K, Spiker DG, Zimmer B, Marin RS, Nelson J, Martin D, Morycz R. Sleep apnea in Alzheimer's dementia: Correlation with mental deterioration. *J Clin Psychiatry* 1985; 46(7):257–261.

Robakis NK, Wisniewski HM, Jenkins EC, Devine-Gage EA, Houck GE, Yao X-L, Ramakrishna N, Wolfe G, Silverman WP, Brown WT. Chromosome 21q21 sublocalisation of gene encoding beta-amyloid peptide in cerebral vessels and neuritic (senile) plaques of people with Alzheimer disease and Down syndrome. *Lancet* 1987; 1(8529):384–385.

Robb S. Exercise treatment for wandering behavior. Paper presented at the 38th annual scientific meeting of the Gerontological Society of America, New Orleans, 1985.

Robinson B, Thurnher M. Taking care of aged parents: A family cycle transition. *Gerontologist* 1979; 19(6):586–593.

Roehrs T, Zorick F, Sicklesteel J, Wittig R, Roth T. Age-related sleep–wake disorders at a sleep disorder center. *J Am Geriatr Soc* 1983; 31(6):364–370.

Roehrs T, Conway W, Wittig R, Zorick F, Sicklesteel J, Roth T. Sleep–wake complaints in patients with sleep-related respiratory disturbances. *Am Rev Respir Dis* 1985; 132(3):520–523.

Rogers JD, Brogan D, Mirra SS. The nucleus basalis of Meynert in neurological disease: A quantitative morphological study. *Ann Neurol* 1985; 17(2):163–170.

Ron MA, Toone BK, Garralda ME, Lishman WA. Diagnostic accuracy in pre-senile dementia. *Br J Psychiatry* 1979; 134:161–168.

Roose SP, Glassman AH, Siris SG, Walsh BT, Bruno RL, Wright LB. Comparison of imipramine and nortriptyline induced orthostatic hypotension: A meaningful difference. *J Clin Psychopharmacol* 1981; 1(5):316–319.

Rose DP, Randall ZC. Reassessment of tryptophan metabolism in breast cancer five years after an initial study. *Clin Chim Acta* 1973; 45(1):33–36.

Rosenthal NP, Keesey J, Crandall B, Brown WJ. Familial neurological disease associated with spongiform encephalopathy. *Arch Neurol* 1976; 33(4):252–259.

Rossi GF. The neural circuitry of sleep. In MH Chase (ed.), *The Sleeping Brain Vol. 1: Perspectives in the Brain Sciences.* [Proceedings of the Symposium of the First International Congress of The Association for the Psychophysiological Study of Sleep, Bruges, Belgium.] Los Angeles: Brain Research Institute, 1972, pp. 85–144.

Roth M, Tomlinson BE, Blessed G. The relationship between quantitative measures of dementia and of degenerative changes in the cerebral grey matter of elderly subjects. *Proc Roy Soc Med* 1967; 60(3):254–258.

Roth M. The psychiatric disorders of later life. *Psychiatry Annals* 1976; 6(9):57–101.

Roth M, Iverson LL (eds.). Alzheimer's disease and related disorders. *Br Med Bull* 1986; 42(1):1–116.

Rubenstein LZ, Josephson KR, Wieland GD, English PA, Sayre JA, Kane RL. Effectiveness of a geriatric evaluation unit. A randomized clinical trial. *N Engl J Med* 1984; 311(26):1664–1670.

Sainsbury P, Grad de Alarcon J. The psychiatrist and the geriatric patient: The effects of community care on the family of the geriatric patient. *J Geriatr Psychiatry* 1970; 4(1):23–41.

Salzman C. A primer on geriatric psychopharmacology. *Am J Psychiatry* 1982; 139(1):67–74.

Salzman C, Shader RI, Greenblatt DJ, Harmatz JS. Long versus short half-life benzodiazepines in the elderly. Kinetics and clinical effects of diazepam and oxazepam. *Arch Gen Psychiatry* 1983; 40(3):293–297.

Salzman C. Treatment of anxiety. In C Salzman (ed.), *Clinical Geriatric Psychopharmacology*. New York: McGraw-Hill, Inc., 1984, pp. 132–148.

Salzman C, van der Kolk B. Treatment of depression. In C Salzman (ed.), *Clinical Geriatric Psychopharmacology*. New York: McGraw-Hill, Inc., 1984, pp. 77–115.

Sanders JF. Evaluation of oxazepam and placebo in emotionally disturbed aged patients. *Geriatrics* 1965; 20:739–746.

Sanford JR. Tolerance of debility in elderly dependents by supporters at home: Its significance for hospital practice. *Br Med J* 1975; 3(5981):471–473.

Saskin P, Spielman AJ, Jelin MA, Thorpy MJ. Sleep restriction therapy for insomnia: A six month follow-up. *Sleep Research* 1984; 13–163.

Schafer SC. Modifying the environment. *Geriatric Nursing* 1985; 6(3):157–159.

Schaie KW. What can we learn from the longitudinal study of adult psychological development? In KW Schaie (ed.), *Longitudinal Studies of Adult Psychological Development*. New York: Guilford Press, 1983, pp. 1–19.

Schwab M, Rader J, Doan J. Relieving the anxiety and fear in dementia. *Journal of Gerontological Nursing* 1985; 11(5):8–15.

Scitovsky AA, Capron AM. Medical care at the end of life: The interaction of economics and ethics. *Annu Rev Public Health* 1986; 7:59–75.

Seager CP. Chlorpromazine in treatment of elderly psychotic women. *Br Med J* 1955; 1:882–885.

Selkoe DJ, Bell DS, Podlisny MB, Price DL, Cork LC. Conservation of brain amyloid proteins in aged mammals and humans with Alzheimer's disease. *Science* 1987; 235(4791):873–877.

Shader RI, Greenblatt DJ. Management of anxiety in the elderly: The balance between therapeutic and adverse effects. *J Clin Psychiatry* 1982; 43(9, Pt 2):8–18.

Shanas E. Social myth as hypothesis: The case of the family relations of old people. *Gerontologist* 1979a; 19(1):3–9.

Shanas E. The family as a social support system in old age. *Gerontologist* 1979b; 19(2):169–174.

Shanas E. Older people and their families: The new pioneers. *Journal of Marriage and the Family* 1980; 42(1):9–15.

Sheikh JI, Yesavage JA. Geriatric Depression Scale (GDS). Recent evidence and development of a shorter version. *Clinical Gerontology* 1986;5(1–2):165–173.

Shindelman LW, Horowitz A, Dobrof R. Reciprocity and affection: Past influences on current caregiving. Paper presented at the 34th annual meeting of the Gerontological Society of America. Toronto, Canada, 1981.

Shraberg D. The myth of pseudodementia: Depression and the aging brain. *Am J Psychiatry* 1978; 135(5):601–603.

Sim M, Sussman I. Alzheimer's disease: Its natural history and differential diagnosis. *J Nerv Ment Dis* 1962; 135(6):489–499.

Smallwood RG, Vitiello MV, Giblin EC, Prinz PN. Sleep apnea: Relationship to age, sex, and Alzheimer's dementia. *Sleep* 1983; 6(1):16–22.

Smith B. Effect of irritant purgatives on the myenteric plexus in man and the mouse. *Gut* 1968; 9:139–143.

Smith B. The neuropathology of the alimentary tract. London: Edward Arnold Publishers Ltd., 1972.

Smith JM, Baldessarini RJ. Changes in prevalence, severity and recovery in tardive dyskinesia with age. *Arch Gen Psychiatry* 1980; 37(12):1368–1373.

Smith PL, Gold AR, Meyers DA, Haponik EF, Bleecker ER. Weight loss in mildly to moderately obese patients with obstructive sleep apnea. *Ann Intern Med* 1985; 103(6, Pt 1):850–855.

Smith RC, Vroulis G, Johnson R, Morgan R. Comparison of therapeutic response to long-term treatment with lecithin versus piracetam plus lecithin in patients with Alzheimer's disease. *Psychopharmacol Bull* 1984; 20(3):542–545.

Smith RG. Fecal incontinence. *J Am Geriatr Soc* 1983; 31(11):694–697.

Snow SS, Wells CE. Case studies in neuropsychiatry: Diagnosis and treatment of coexistent dementia and depression. *J Clin Psychiatry* 1981; 42(11):439–441.

Soininen H, Koskinen T, Helkala EL, Pigache R, Reikkinen PJ. Treatment of Alzheimer's disease with a synthetic ACTH 4-9 analog. *Neurology* 1985; 35(9):1348–1351.

Soldo BJ. The dependency squeeze on middle-aged women. Paper presented at meeting of the Secretary's Advisory Committee on Rights and Responsibilities of Women. Department of Health and Human Services, Washington, DC: 1980.

Soldo BJ, Myllyluoma J. Caregivers who live with dependent elderly. *Gerontologist* 1983; 23(6):605–611.

Somers AR. Long-term care for the elderly and disabled: A new health priority. *N Engl J Med* 1982; 307(4):221–226.

Southwell PR, Evans CR, Hunt JN. Effect of a hot milk drink on movements during sleep. *Br Med J* 1972; 2:429–431.

Spielman AJ, Saskin P, Thorpy MJ. Sleep restriction treatment of insomnia. *Sleep Research* 1983; 12:286.

Spinweber CL, Ursin R, Hilbert RP, Hildebrand RL. L-tryptophan: Effects on daytime sleep latency and the waking EEG. *Electroencephalogr Clin Neurophysiol* 1983; 55(6):652–661.

St. George-Hyslop PH, Tanzi RE, Polinsky RJ, Haines JL, Nee L, Watkins PC, Myers RH, Feldman RG, Pollen D, Drachman D, Growdon J, Bruni A, Foncin J-F, Salmon D, Frommelt P, Amaducci L, Sorbi S, Piacentini S, Stewart GD, Hobbs WJ, Conneally PM, Gusella JF. The genetic defect causing familial Alzheimer's disease maps on chromosome 21. *Science* 1987; 235(4791):885–890.

Steel K. Iatrogenic disease on a medical service. *J Am Geriatr Soc* 1984; 32(6):445–449.

Steele C, Lucas MJ, Tune L. An approach to the management of dementia syndromes. *Johns Hopkins Medical Journal* 1982; 151(6):362–368.

Stoller EP, Earl LL. Help with activities of everyday life: Sources of support for the noninstitutionalized elderly. *Gerontologist* 1983; 23(1):64–70.

Stoller EP. Parental caregiving by adult children. *Journal of Marriage and the Family* 1983; 45(4):851–858.

Stone R, Casserata GL, Sangl J. Caregivers of the frail elderly: A national profile. *Gerontologist* (in press).

Storandt M, Botwinick J, Danzinger WL, Berg L, Hughes CP. Psychometric differentiation of mild senile dementia of the Alzheimer type. *Arch Neurol* 1984, 41(5):497–499.

Stotsky B. Multicenter study comparing thioridazine with diazepam and placebo in elderly, non-psychotic patients with emotional and behavioral disorders. *Clin Ther* 1984; 6(4):546–559.

Strayhorn JM Jr, Nash JL. Severe neurotoxicity despite "therapeutic" serum lithium levels. *Diseases of the Nervous System* 1977; 38(2):107–111.

Suber DG, Tabor WJ. Withholding of life-sustaining treatment from the terminally ill incompetent patient: Who decides? Parts I, II. *JAMA* 1982; 248(18):2250–2251; 248(19):2431–2432.

Sugerman AA, Williams BH, Adlerstein AM. Haloperidol in the psychiatric disorders of old age. *Am J Psychiatry* 1964; 120:1190–1192.

Sulkava R, Haltia M, Paetau A, Wikstrom J, Palo J. Accuracy of clinical diagnosis in primary degenerative dementia: Correlation with neuropathological findings. *J Neurol Neurosurg Psychiatry* 1983; 46(1):9–13.

Sullivan ES, Corman ML, Devroede G, Rudd WWH, Schuster MM. Symposium: Anal incontinence. *Dis Colon Rectum* 1982; 25(2):90–107.

Summers WK, Viesselman JO, Marsh GM, Candelora K. Use of THA in treatment of Alzheimer-like dementia: Pilot study in twelve patients. *Biol Psychiatry* 1981; 16(2):145–153.

Summers WK, Majovski LV, Marsh GM, Tachiki K, Kling A. Oral tetrahydroaminoacridine in long-term treatment of senile dementia, Alzheimer type. *N Engl J Med* 1986; 315(20):1241–1245.

Sunderland T, Tariot PN, Mueller EA, Murphy DL, Weingartner H, Cohen RM. Cognitive and behavioral sensitivity to scopolamine in Alzheimer patients and controls. *Psychopharmacol Bull* 1985; 21(3):676–679.

Sussman MB. Relationships of adult children with their parents in the United States. In E Shanas & GF Streib (eds.), *Social Structure and the Family: Generational Relations*. Englewood Cliffs, N.J.: Prentice-Hall, 1965, pp. 62–92.

Tanzi RE, Gusella JF, Watkins PC, Bruns GAP, St. George Hyslop P, Van Keuren ML, Patterson D, Pagan S, Kurnit DM, Neve RL. Amyloid beta protein gene: cDNA, mRNA distribution, and genetic linkage near the Alzheimer locus. *Science* 1987; 235(4791):880–884.

Tariot PN, Sunderland T, Weingartner H, Murphy DL, Cohen MR, Cohen RM. Low- and high-dose naloxone in dementia of the Alzheimer type. *Psychopharmacol Bull* 1985; 21(3):680–682.

Terry RD, Davies P. Dementia of the Alzheimer type. *Annu Rev Neurosci* 1980; 3:77–95.

Tewfik GI, Jain VK, Harcup M, Magowan S. Effectiveness of various tranquilizers in the management of senile restlessness. *Gerontologia Clinica* 1970; 12(6):351–359.

Thal LJ, Fuld PA, Masur DM, Sharpless NS. Oral physostigmine and lecithin improve memory in Alzheimer's disease. *Ann Neurol* 1983; 13(5):491–496.

Thoman M. Role of interleukin-2 in the age-related impairment of immune function. *J Am Geriatr Soc* 1985; 33(11):781–787.

Thomas, L. On the problem of dementia. *Discover*. August, 1981, pp. 34–36.

Thomas, L. The Lasker Award: Four Decades of Scientific Medical Progress. New York: Albert and Mary Lasker Foundation, 1985, pp. 1–7.

Tinklenberg JR, Thornton JE. Neuropeptides in geriatric psychopharmacology. *Psychopharmacol Bull* 1983; 19(2):198–211.

Tobin AJ. Alzheimer's disease: Enter molecular biology. *Alzheimer Disease and Associated Disorders* 1987; 1:69.

Tobin SS, Kulys R. The family and services. In C. Eisdorfer (ed.), *Annual Review of Gerontology & Geriatrics,* Vol 1. New York: Springer Publishing Co., 1980, pp. 370–399.

Torrey BB. Sharing increasing costs on declining income: The visible dilemma of the invisible aged. *Milbank Mem Fund Q* 1985; 63(2):377–394.

Townsend P. The effects of family structure on the likelihood of admission to an institution in old age: The application of a general theory. In E. Shanas & GF Streib (eds.), *Social Structure and the Family: Generational Relations.* Englewood Cliffs, N.J.: Prentice-Hall, 1965, pp. 163–187.

Treas J. Family support systems for the aged: Some social and demographic considerations. *Gerontologist* 1977; 17(6):486–491.

Troll LE. The family of later life: A decade review. *Journal of Marriage and the Family* 1971; 33(2):263–290.

U.S. Department of Health and Human Services *Differential Diagnosis of Dementing Disease.* National Institutes of Health Consensus Development Conference Statement, Vol. 6,(11). Washington, DC: National Institutes of Health, 1987a.

Uhlmann RF, Larson EB, Koepsell TD. Hearing impairment and cognitive decline in senile dementia of the Alzheimer's type. *J Am Geriatr Soc* 1986; 34(3):207–210.

University of Michigan. *The Veterans Administration and Dementia: Recommendations for Patient Care, Research and Training, by an International Work Group.* Ann Arbor: Institute of Gerontology, University of Michigan, 1985.

U.S. Department of Health and Human Services Task Force on Alzheimer's Disease. *Alzheimer's Disease.* (ADM-84-1323). Washington, DC: U.S. Government Printing Office, 1984a.

U.S. Department of Health and Human Services. *Alzheimer's Disease: A Scientific Guide for Health Practitioners* (NIH-84-2251). Bethesda, MD: National Institutes of Health, 1984b.

U.S. Department of Health and Human Services. *Report on Education and Training in Geriatrics and Gerontology.* Washington, DC: National Institute on Aging administrative document, 1984c.

U.S. Department of Health and Human Services. *Sixth Report to Council on Program.* Washington, DC: National Institute on Aging administrative document, 1984d.

U.S. Department of Health and Human Services. Personnel for Health Needs of the Elderly Through the Year 2020. Washington, DC: National Institutes of Health, 1987b.

U.S. General Accounting Office. *Medicaid and Nursing Home Care: Cost In-*

creases and the Need for Services Are Creating Problems for the States and the Elderly. Washington, DC: U.S. General Accounting Office, 1984.

U.S. Veterans Administration. *Caring for the Older Veteran.* Washington, DC: Veterans Administration, 1984.

U.S. Veterans Administration. *Dementia. Guidelines for Diagnosis and Treatment.* (Prepared by the Office of Geriatrics and Extended Care, Department of Medicine and Surgery.) Washington, DC: Veterans Administration, 1985.

van Loveren-Huyben CM, Engelaar HF, Hermans MB, van der Bom JA, Leering C, Munnichs JM. Double-blind clinical and psychological study of ergoloid mesylates (Hydergine) in subjects with senile mental deterioration. *J Am Geriatr Soc* 1984; 32(8):584–588.

Veatch RM. *A Theory of Medical Ethics.* New York: Basic Books, 1981.

Venn RD. The Sandoz Clinical Assessment-Geriatric (SCAG) Scale. A general purpose psychogeriatric rating scale. *Gerontology* 1983; 29(3):185–198.

Verwoerdt A. Individual psychotherapy in senile dementia. In NE Miller & GD Cohen (eds.), *Clinical Aspects of Alzheimer's Disease and Senile Dementia,* Vol 15: *Aging.* New York: Raven Press, 1981, pp. 187–208.

Vitiello MV, Bokon JA, Kukull WA, Muniz RL, Smallwood RG, Prinz PN. Rapid eye movement sleep measures of Alzheimer's-type dementia patients and optimally healthy aged individuals. *Biol Psychiatry* 1984; 19(5):721–734.

Wald A. Biofeedback therapy for fecal incontinence. *Ann Intern Med* 1981; 95(2):146–149.

Wanzer SH, Adelstein SJ, Cranford RE, Federman DD, Hook ED, Moertel CG, Safar P, Stone A, Taussig HB, van Eys J. The physician's responsibility toward hopelessly ill patients. *N Engl J Med* 1984; 310(15):955–959.

Warren JW, Sobal J, Tenney JH, Hoopes JM, Damon D, Levenson S, DeForge BR, Muncie HL Jr. Informed consent by proxy. An issue in research with elderly patients. *N Engl J Med* 1986; 315(18):1124–1128.

Wechsler D. A standardized memory scale for clinical use. *J Psychol* 1945; 19:87–95.

Wechsler D. *Wechsler Adult Intelligence Scale Manual.* New York: Psychological Corporation, 1955.

Wechsler D. *WAIS-R Manual.* New York: Psychological Corporation, 1981.

Weiner IH, Weiner HL. Nocturnal leg muscle cramps. *JAMA* 1980; 244(20):2332–2333.

Weingartner H, Kaye W, Smallberg SA, Ebert MH, Gillin JC, Sitaram N. Memory failures in progressive idiopathic dementia. *J Abnorm Psychol* 1981; 90(3):187–196.

Weingartner H, Silberman E. Models of cognitive impairment: Cognitive changes in depression. *Psychopharmacol Bull* 1982; 18(2):27–42.

Weingartner H. Drugs that facilitate cognitive processes: Characterizing the response. *Drug Development Research* 1985; 5(1):25–38.

Weintraub S, Mesulam MM, Auty R, Baratz R, Cholakos BN, Kapust L, Ransil B, Tellers JG, Albert MS, LoCastro S, Moss M. Lecithin in the treatment of Alzheimer's disease [letter]. *Arch Neurol* 1983; 40(8):527–528.

Weissert WG. Seven reasons why it is so difficult to make community based long-term care cost effective. *Journal of Health Services Research* 1985; 20:423–433.

Wells CE. Pseudodementia. *Am J Psychiatry* 1979; 136(7):895–900.

Wettstein A, Spiegel R. Clinical trials with the cholinergic drug RS 86 in Alzheimer's disease (AD) and senile dementia of the Alzheimer type (SDAT). *Psychopharmacology* (Berlin) 1984; 84(4):572–573.

Whall AL, Conklin C. Why a psychogeriatric unit? *J Psychosoc Nurs Ment Health Serv* 1985; 23(5):23–27.

Whalley LJ, Carothers AD, Collyer S, De Mey R, Frackiewicz A. A study of familial factors in Alzheimer's disease. *Br J Psychiatry* 1982; 140:249–256.

Whitehouse PJ, Price DL, Clark AW, Coyle JT, DeLong MR. Alzheimer's disease: Evidence for selective loss of cholinergic neurons in the nucleus basalis. *Ann Neurol* 1981; 10(2):122–126.

Wilder DE, Teresi JA, Bennett RG. Family burden and dementia. In R Mayeux & WG Rosen (eds.), *The Dementias*, Vol. 38: *Advances in Neurology*. New York: Raven Press, 1983, pp. 239–251.

Wilkin D, Jolley DJ. Mental and physical impairment in the elderly in hospital and residential care. 1. [occasional paper]. *Nursing Times* 1978; 74(29):117–120.

Williams KH, Goldstein G. Cognitive and affective response to lithium in patients with organic brain syndrome. *Am J Psychiatry* 1979; 136(6):800–803.

Wilson RS, Bacon LD, Fox JH, Kaszniak AW. Primary memory and secondary memory in dementia of the Alzheimer type. *Journal of Clinical Neuropsychology* 1983; 5(4):337–344.

Wincor MZ. Insomnia and the new benzodiazepines. *Clin Pharm* 1982; 1(5):425–432.

Winograd CH. Long-term care: Mental status tests and the capacity for self-care. *J Am Geriatr Soc* 1984; 32(1):49–55.

Winograd CH, Jarvik LF. Physician management of the demented patient. *J Am Geriatr Soc* 1986; 34(4):295–308.

Wisniewski KE, Jervis GA, Moretz RC, Wisniewski HM. Alzheimer neurofibrillary tangles in diseases other than senile and presenile dementia. *Ann Neurol* 1979; 5(3):288–294.

Wisniewski KE, Wisniewski HM, Wen GY. Occurrence of neuropathological changes and dementia of Alzheimer's disease in Down's syndrome. *Ann Neurol* 1985; 17(3):278–282.

Wolanin MO, Phillips LR. Care of the patient with a true dementia. In MO Wolanin & LR Phillips (eds.), *Confusion: Prevention and Care*. St. Louis: CV Mosby Co., 1981, pp. 319–349.

Wolanin MO. Confusion and disorientation. In B Steffl (ed.), *Handbook of Gerontological Nursing*. New York: Van Nostrand-Reinhold Co., 1984, pp. 119–134.

Wolozin BL, Pruchnicki A, Dickson DW, Davies P. A neuronal antigen in the brains of Alzheimer patients. *Science* 1986; 232(4750):648–650.

Wong CW, Quaranta V, Glenner GG. Neuritic plaques and cerebrovascular amyloid in Alzheimer's disease are antigenically related. *Proc Natl Acad Sci USA* 1985; 82(23):8729–8732.

Wurtman R. Alzheimer's disease. *Sci Am* 1985a; 252(1):62–66, 71–74.

Wurtman R. Activation of neurotransmitters in the brain: Strategies in the treatment of AD/SDAT. In CG Gottfries (ed.), *Normal Aging, Alzheimer's Disease and Senile Dementia*. Brussels: Èdition de l'Université de Bruxelles, 1985b, pp. 275–280.

Yarmesch M, Sheafor M. The decision to restrain. *Geriatric Nursing* 1984; 5(6):242–244.

Yerby MS, Sundsten JW, Larson EB, Wu SA, Sumi SM. A new method of measuring brain atrophy. The effect of aging in its application for diagnosing dementia. *Neurology* 1985; 35(9):1316–1320.

Yesavage JA, Tinklenberg JR, Hollister LE, Berger PA. Vasodilators in senile dementias: A review of the literature. *Arch Gen Psychiatry* 1979; 36(2):220–223.

Zarit SH, Reever KE, Bach-Peterson J. Relatives of the impaired elderly: Correlates of feelings of burden. *Gerontologist* 1980; 20(6):649–655.

Zarit SH, Zarit JM. Families under stress: Interventions for caregivers of senile dementia patients. *Psychotherapy: Theory, Research and Practice* 1982; 19(4):461–471.

Zarit SH, Orr NK, Zarit JM. *The Hidden Victims of Alzheimer's Disease: Families Under Stress.* New York: New York University Press, 1985.

Zarit SH, Anthony CR. Interventions with dementia patients and their families. In JE Birren, MLM Gilhooly & SH Zarit (eds.), *The Senile Dementias. Policy and Management.* Englewood Cliffs, NJ: Prentice-Hall (1986).

Zimmer AH, Sainer JS. Strengthening the family as an informal support for the aged: Two service strategies-Implications for social policy and planning. Paper presented at the 31st annual meeting of the Gerontological Society, Dallas, TX, 1978.

Zung W. A self-rating depression scale. *Arch Gen Psychiatry*, 1965; 12:63–70.

Resources*

Organizations

Administration on Aging (AOA)
330 Independence Avenue, S.W.   (202) 245-0724
Washington, DC 20201

A governmental agency that acts as advocate for the elderly and serves as
the principal agency for implementing programs of the Older Americans
Act.

Alzheimer's Disease and Related Disorders Association (ADRDA)
70 East Lake Street   (800) 621-0379, in Illinois (800) 572-6037
Chicago, IL 60601-5997

A voluntary national health organization of Alzheimer family members
with local chapters throughout the country dedicated to easing the burden and finding the cure for Alzheimer's Disease and related disorders.
This mission is carried out through research, education, chapter formation, advocacy and patient and family service.

American Association for Geriatric Psychiatry (AAGP)
P.O. Box 376A   (301) 220-0952
Greenbelt, MD 20770

An association of over 800 psychiatrists throughout the United States
who specialize in treating mental disorders of the older patient.

American Association of Retired Persons (AARP)
1909 K Street, N.W.   (202) 872-4700
Washington, DC 20049

A national organization of 24 million older Americans (not all retired)
that provides a wide range of member benefits and service programs.

*Inclusion in this list is not intended as an endorsement of any given organization or
publication.

Familial Alzheimer's Disease Research Foundation (FADRF)
8177 S. Harvard, Suite 114   (918) 493-8476 or 481-6100
Tulsa, OK 74137

A foundation that primarily facilitates worldwide research in familial Alzheimer's disease in addition to developing a research center and diagnostic clinic in Tulsa.

Publications (see also reference list, pp. 221)

Agenda to Action: The Aging Network Responses to Alzheimer's Disease. New York: New York City Department for the Aging and the Brookdale Foundation, 1986.

A directory and summary of current services offered to Alzheimer's disease patients and families by 244 State and Area Agencies on Aging in 46 states. Included are specially designed Alzheimer programs at the community level and state efforts such as task forces and study commissions to recommend policy. It also lists 12 national demonstration projects of the Federal Administration on Aging, and the collaborative activities of State offices and Area Agencies on Aging with the Alzheimer's Disease and Related Disorder Association, other government agencies, medical centers, and private industry.

Alzheimer Disease and Associated Disorders—An International Journal.
Western Geriatric Research Institute
P.O. Box 368
Lawrence, Kansas 66044

This journal is an international medium for publication of authoritative and original contributions with primary emphasis on Alzheimer's disease and associated disorders. There are also reports on legislative actions as well as pending legislation which could have an impact on research funding, brief accounts of transactions at various national conferences, and abstracts of current relevant literature.

American Hospital Formulary Service: Drug Information 87. Bethesda, MD: American Society of Hospital Pharmacists, 1987.

A valuable resource for information regarding drug indications, actions, and side effects, and drug-drug, drug-disease interactions.

The American Journal of Alzheimer's Care and Related Disorders and Research.
470 Boston Post Road   (617) 899-2702
Weston, MA 02193

A publication dedicated to bringing the latest information from the medical, scientific, research, caregiving, legal and public policy areas together all in one source for Alzheimer professionals, paraprofessionals and caregivers. Conferences, newsbriefs, and reviews of the newest publications and films are also featured.

Caring: A Family Guide to Managing the Alzheimer's Patient at Home. New York: New York City Department for the Aging, 1987.

A 100 page illustrated manual detailing step-by-step guidelines for managing the patient through the various stages of this progressive disease with up-to-date, recommended practices by medical experts and professional care providers. Topics include: how to communicate with the Alzheimer patient; creating a safe environment; exercise and movement; and activities of daily living.

Consensus Development Conference Statement: Differential Diagnosis of Dementing Disease (July, 1987). Bethesda, MD : NIH, 1987.

To assess the current state of knowledge about the differential diagnosis of the dementias, NIH convened a consensus development conference. A consensus statement was published on the questions: (1) What is dementia? (2) What are the dementing diseases? (3) What should be included in the initial evaluation of dementia? (4) What diagnostic tests should be performed? (5) What are the priorities for research?

Generations. MK Aronson and LF Jarvik. Winter 1984. Vol. 9(2), 72 pp. Western Gerontological Society. San Francisco, CA.

The entire issue is devoted to an update on Alzheimer's disease. Available in libraries and from ADRDA and the Western Gerontological Society, 833 Market St., Room 516, San Francisco, CA 94103.

Generations. MK Aronson and R Katzman. Fall 1982, Vol. 7(1), 64pp. Western Gerontological Society, San Francisco, CA.

The entire issue of this quarterly publication was devoted to the subject of Alzheimer's disease. Available only in libraries.

Losing a Million Minds: Confronting the Tragedy of Alzheimer's Disease and other Dementias. U.S. Office of Technology Assessment, Washington, DC: GPO. 1987.

This book is a compendium of biomedical and health services research related to Alzheimer's disease and provides a valuable resource for professionals and non-professionals.

Drug Index

The drug index is an alphabetical listing of drugs that are mentioned in this book. Page references are provided for generic drugs only. Many of the drugs indexed below are brand names of generic drugs. Brand names and generic names are cross referenced; see generic names for page number.

Inclusion in this index is not intended as an endorsement of any given product.

Dio-Sul, *see* Dioctyl sodium sulfosuccinate (DSS)
Diphen, *see* Diphenhydramine
Diphenacen, *see* Diphenhydramine
Diphenatol, *see* Diphenoxylate
Diphenhydramine, 18
    Allerdryl 50; AllerMax; Belix; Bena-D; Benadryl; Benadryl Kapseals; Benahist; Ben-Allergin; Benaphen; Benoject; Benylin; Bydramine; Compoz; Diahist; Dihydrex; Diphen; Diphenacen; Dormarex 2; Fenylhist; Hydril; Hyrexin; Miles Nervine Nighttime Sleep Aid; Nordryl; Nytol; Sleep-Eze 3; Sleepinal Night-time Sleep Aid; Sominex 2; Surfadil; Tusstat; Valdrene; Wehdryl
Diphenoxylate, 34
    Diphenatol; Diphenoxylate with Atropine Sulfate; Lofene; Logen; Lomanate; Lomotil; Lonox; Lo-Trol; Low-Quel; Nor-Mil; SK-Diphenoxylate
Disanthrol, *see* Dioctyl sodium sulfosuccinate (DSS)
Disolan, *see* Dioctyl sodium sulfosuccinate (DSS)
Disolan Forte, *see* Dioctyl sodium sulfosuccinate (DSS)
Disolan with Docusate Sodium, *see* Phenolphthalein
Disonate, *see* Dioctyl sodium sulfosuccinate (DSS)
Disoplex, *see* Dioctyl sodium sulfosuccinate (DSS), Psyllium preparations
Di-Sosul, *see* Dioctyl sodium sulfosuccinate (DSS)
Docusate Sodium, *see* Dioctyl sodium sulfosuccinate (DSS)
Docusate sodium with casanthranol, *see* Dioctyl sodium sulfosuccinate (DSS)
DOK, *see* Dioctyl sodium sulfosuccinate (DSS)
Dolprn #3, *see* Magnesium hydroxide
Donnagel, *see* Scopolamine hydrobromide
Dorbantyl, *see* Dioctyl sodium sulfosuccinate (DSS)

Dorbantyl Forte, *see* Dioctyl sodium sulfosuccinate (DSS)
Dormarex 2, *see* Diphenhydramine
Doss, *see* Dioctyl sodium sulfosuccinate (DSS)
Doss 300, *see* Dioctyl sodium sulfosuccinate (DSS)
Dotazone, *see* Trazodone
Doxepin, 9, 21, 63
    Adapin; Saxapin; Sinequan
Doxinate, *see* Dioctyl sodium sulfosuccinate (DSS)
Dr. Caldwell Senna Laxative, *see* Senna concentrates
Drocarbil, *see* Arecoline
D-S-S, *see* Dioctyl sodium sulfosuccinate (DSS)
D-S-S Plus, *see* Dioctyl sodium sulfosuccinate (DSS)
Dulcolax, *see* Bisacodyl
Duosol, *see* Dioctyl sodium sulfosuccinate (DSS)
Durapam, *see* Flurazepam
Duvoid, *see* Bethanechol chloride

Effer-Syllium, *see* Psyllium preparations
Elavil, *see* Amitriptyline
Emitrip, *see* Amitriptyline
Endep, *see* Amitriptyline
Enovil, *see* Amitriptyline
Ergoloid mesylates, 9, 73, 74, 75
    Deapril ST; Gerimal; Hydergine; Hydergine LC; Hydro-Ergoloid; Hydro-Ergot; Hydroloid-G; Niloric; Uni-Gine
Eskalith, *see* Lithium (carbonate)
Eskalith CR, *see* Lithium (carbonate)
Espotabs, *see* Phenolphthalein
Etiracetam, 75
Etrafon, *see* Amitriptyline, Perphenazine
Evac-Q-Kit, *see* Phenolphthalein
Evac-Q-Kwik, *see* Phenolphthalein, Bisacodyl
Evac-U-Gen, *see* Phenolphthalein
Evac-U-Lax, *see* Phenolphthalein
Ex-Lax, *see* Phenolphthalein
Ex-Lax Extra Gentle, *see* Dioctyl sodium sulfosuccinate (DSS), Phenolphthalein

Index